The Pocket Guide to
Cornea

T0131093

Ophthalmology Pocket Guides
Series

SERIES EDITOR, RICHARD L. LINDSTROM

The Pocket Guide to
Cornea

EDITORS

Terry Kim, MD
Professor of Ophthalmology
Duke University School of Medicine
Chief, Cornea and External Disease Division
Director, Refractive Surgery Service
Duke University Eye Center
Durham, North Carolina

Melissa B. Daluvoy, MD
Assistant Professor of Ophthalmology
Duke University School of Medicine
Cornea, Refractive and External Disease Fellowship Director
Duke University Eye Center
Durham, North Carolina

ASSOCIATE EDITORS

Michelle J. Kim, MD
Clinical Associate
Duke University School of Medicine
Cornea, Refractive and External Disease Fellowship Director
Duke University Eye Center
Durham, North Carolina

Nambi Nallasamy, MD
Cornea, External Disease, and Refractive Surgery
Assistant Professor of Ophthalmology and Visual Science
University of Michigan, Kellogg Eye Center
Ann Arbor, Michigan

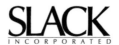

SLACK
INCORPORATED

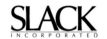

SLACK INCORPORATED

Senior Vice President: Stephanie Arasim Portnoy
Vice President, Editorial: Jennifer Kilpatrick
Vice President, Marketing: Michelle Gatt
Acquisitions Editor: Brien Cummings
Managing Editor: Allegra Tiver
Creative Director: Thomas Cavallaro
Cover Artist: Ryan Davis
Project Editor: Joseph Lowery

SLACK Incorporated
6900 Grove Road
Thorofare, NJ 08086 USA
856-848-1000   Fax: 856-848-6091
www.Healio.com/books
© 2019 by SLACK Incorporated

The procedures and practices described in this publication should be implemented in a manner consistent with the professional standards set for the circumstances that apply in each specific situation. Every effort has been made to confirm the accuracy of the information presented and to correctly relate generally accepted practices. The authors, editors, and publisher cannot accept responsibility for errors or exclusions or for the outcome of the material presented herein. There is no expressed or implied warranty of this book or information imparted by it. Care has been taken to ensure that drug selection and dosages are in accordance with currently accepted/recommended practice. Off-label uses of drugs may be discussed. Due to continuing research, changes in government policy and regulations, and various effects of drug reactions and interactions, it is recommended that the reader carefully review all materials and literature provided for each drug, especially those that are new or not frequently used. Some drugs or devices in this publication have clearance for use in a restricted research setting by the Food and Drug and Administration or FDA. Each professional should determine the FDA status of any drug or device prior to use in their practice.

Any review or mention of specific companies or products is not intended as an endorsement by the author or publisher.

SLACK Incorporated uses a review process to evaluate submitted material. Prior to publication, educators or clinicians provide important feedback on the content that we publish. We welcome feedback on this work.

Library of Congress Cataloging-in-Publication Data
Names: Kim, Terry, author. | Daluvoy, Melissa B., author.
Title: The pocket guide to cornea / Terry Kim, Melissa B. Daluvoy.
Description: Thorofare, NJ : SLACK Incorporated, [2019] | Includes
  bibliographical references and index. |
Identifiers: LCCN 2019010828 (print) | LCCN 2019011279 (ebook) | ISBN
  9781630914196 (Epub) | ISBN 9781630914202 (Web) | ISBN 9781630914189 (pbk.)
Subjects: | MESH: Cornea | Corneal Diseases | Handbook
Classification: LCC RE336 (ebook) | LCC RE336 (print) | NLM WW 39 | DDC
  617.7/19--dc23
LC record available at https://lccn.loc.gov/2019010828

Printed in the United States of America.

Last digit is print number: 10   9   8   7   6   5   4   3   2   1

DEDICATION

To my wife, Ellie, and my children, Ashley and Kayley,
for their never-ending love, support, and understanding.

To my parents, Kyung Hwae and Hyun Sim Kim, for raising me,
educating me, supporting me, and taking care of me.

To all my resident, fellow, and medical student trainees, for
constantly stimulating my mind, inspiring me to be a
better teacher, and keeping me young.

To all of my teachers and mentors, for their valuable guidance
and inspiration, and for giving me professional and personal
goals to strive for as they lead by example.

To all my faculty and colleagues at Duke University, Duke
University School of Medicine, and Duke University Eye Center,
with whom it has been a pleasure and privilege to practice,
research, and collaborate, and who have supported my career.

—Terry Kim, MD

To all my teachers in the past and my colleagues today who
continue to help and teach me everyday.

To all the students, residents, & fellows that have given me the
pleasure of teaching them and to all my patients who have given
me the honor of taking care of them.

Most of all to my family & friends who have always believed in
me, my husband who has always supported me, and to my
children, Terrick & Myla who constantly make me smile!!

—Melissa B. Daluvoy, MD

To my family, friends, Narae Ko, Nikki Fuerst, and all of my
mentors and colleagues who have molded me into
the person I am today.

—Michelle J. Kim, MD

To all my teachers and mentors, who
continue to inspire me to this day.

To my family, whose steadfast support has
made possible everything I do.

—Nambi Nallasamy, MD

Contents

ACKNOWLEDGMENTS

We are fortunate to have so many bright, talented, creative, and curious medical students, residents, fellows, and practitioners in our field who continue to ask intriguing questions and force us to stay current and relevant with our knowledge base. We certainly had this particular group of individuals in mind when we wrote this book, and we would like to acknowledge them here. We hope they find this unique pocket guide on the cornea a useful and well-utilized resource.

Two of our very own trainees, Drs. Michelle J. Kim and Nambi Nallasamy, are actually coeditors of this book. We were so taken by their energy and enthusiasm for this project that we decided to make them coeditors. We would like to take this opportunity to thank them for their contributions to this cornea book. Their tasks included authoring chapter content, gathering photos and references, answering queries, and editing so many versions of our drafts, and we are extremely grateful for all of their efforts. This book is as much theirs as it is ours.

Thirdly, we would also like to recognize the numerous residents and clinicians in both private practice and academic environments that assisted us in reviewing and critiquing the content of this pocket guide book.

In addition, we are extremely grateful to Tony Schiavo and his wonderful and resourceful team at SLACK Incorporated's Health Care Books and Journals division. Their professionalism, guidance, and dedication to this project helped make this book a reality and a success. We would specifically like to thank the following individuals for their assistance and oversight: Joseph Lowery, Allegra Tiver, Dani Malady, and Nathan Quinn.

Last but not certainly not least, we would like to thank our families for allowing us to devote our time and energy toward completing this important and worthwhile project.

—*Terry Kim, MD*
—*Melissa B. Daluvoy, MD*

ABOUT THE EDITORS

Dr. Terry Kim, MD, Professor of Ophthalmology at Duke University Eye Center, received his medical degree from Duke University School of Medicine and completed his residency and chief residency in ophthalmology at Emory Eye Center. He continued with his fellowship training in Cornea, External Disease, and Refractive Surgery at Wills Eye Hospital. He was then recruited to Duke University Eye Center, where he serves as principal and co-investigator on a number of clinical trials and research grants from the National Institutes of Health and other industry sponsors. Dr. Kim was formerly the Director of the Residency Program and Ophthalmology Fellowship Programs and currently serves as Chief of the Cornea and External Disease Division, Director of the Refractive Surgery Service, and Director of the Duke Sports Vision Center.

Dr. Kim's clinical and surgical expertise has resulted in continual annual listings by Best Doctors in America, Best Doctors in North Carolina, and America's Top Ophthalmologists since 2003 as well as featured stories on the Discovery Channel and The Wall Street Journal. He has also been voted by his peers as one of 300 Premier Surgeons in *Ocular Surgery News*, one of the 250 most prominent cataract and intraocular lens surgeons in the country in *Premier Surgeon*, one of the "135 Leading Ophthalmologists in America" in *Becker's ASC Review*, as well as one of the "Top 50 Opinion Leaders" in *Cataract & Refractive Surgery Today*.

His academic accomplishments include over 300 peer-reviewed journal articles, textbook chapters, and scientific abstracts. He is also editor and author of 4 well-respected textbooks on corneal diseases, corneal transplantation, and cataract surgery. Dr. Kim has delivered over 300 invited lectures both nationally and internationally, including numerous named lectureships. He has been the recipient of the Achievement Award and the Senior Achievement Award from the American Academy of

Ophthalmology (AAO) and the American Society of Cataract and Refractive Surgery (ASCRS) Film Festival Award. His clinical and research work has earned him honors and grants from the National Institutes of Health, the Fight for Sight/Research to Prevent Blindness Foundation, the Heed Ophthalmic Foundation, Alcon Laboratories, and Allergan.

Dr. Kim serves on the Executive Committee of ASCRS, the Annual Program Committee of the AAO, and the Executive Committee and Board of Directors of the Cornea Society. He also sits on the Editorial Board for several peer-reviewed journals and trade publications, including *Cornea*, *Journal of Cataract & Refractive Surgery*, *Ocular Surgery News*, *Eyeworld*, *Cataract & Refractive Surgery Today*, *Premier Surgeon*, *Review of Ophthalmology*, and *Advanced Ocular Care*. Dr. Kim serves as Consultant to the Ophthalmic Devices Panel of the FDA, Consultant Ophthalmologist for the Duke Men's Basketball Team, and Consultant to numerous ophthalmic companies.

Melissa B. Daluvoy, MD is an Assistant Professor of Ophthalmology at Duke University Eye Center. She received her medical degree from Thomas Jefferson Medical College and completed her residency in ophthalmology at George Washington University. She then went on to complete a fellowship in cornea and external disease at Wills Eye Institute. She began her career working and teaching residents at the Veterans Affairs Hospital in Washington DC; she then moved to North Carolina and began working at Duke University Eye Center specializing in complex ocular surface disease, high-risk corneal transplants, and pediatric cornea cases. She is Fellowship Director for the cornea department. She also serves as Co-Director of North Carolina's Opening Eyes program for the Special Olympics.

ABOUT THE ASSOCIATE EDITORS

Michelle J. Kim, MD received her medical degree from the University of California, Los Angeles (UCLA). She completed her residency in ophthalmology and a fellowship in cornea, external disease, and refractive surgery at the Duke University Eye Center. She then served as a Clinical Associate at the Duke University Eye Center and now practices in California.

Nambi Nallasamy, MD is a cornea, external disease, and refractive surgery specialist at the University of Michigan Kellogg Eye Center in Ann Arbor, Michigan. Dr. Nallasamy earned his medical degree from Harvard Medical School and the Harvard-MIT Division of Health Sciences and Technology (HST). He completed his residency in ophthalmology at Duke University Eye Center and subsequently completed a cornea, external disease, and refractive surgery fellowship at Bascom Palmer Eye Institute. Dr. Nallasamy is a recipient of the Heed Fellowship for ophthalmologists pursuing research in the visual sciences. In addition to his clinical work, Dr. Nallasamy conducts a research program dedicated to the application of machine learning to clinical informatics, attempting to glean novel insights into disease processes through the use of artificial intelligence.

INTRODUCTION

This book is designed to give ophthalmologists in training as well as general ophthalmologists a concise but complete overview of corneal diseases they may see in clinic. It is meant to be easy to maneuver with images to help solidify learning and help with recognition.

1

Examination and Diagnostic Testing

SLIT-LAMP EXAMINATION

Direct Illumination

The light beam is focused on the area you are examining.

Diffuse Illumination. Use a broad beam with lower intensity and low magnification to give an overview of the cornea and anterior segment (Figure 1-1).

Slit-Lamp Illumination. Use a thin beam to view a section of the cornea. This can be used to closely examine the individual layers of the cornea as well as the presence of cell or flare in the anterior chamber (Figure 1-2. Note central Descemet's detachment and stromal edema).

Indirect Illumination

The light beam is directed to the side or behind the area to be examined.

Kim T, Daluvoy MB.
The Pocket Guide to Cornea (pp 1-10).
© 2019 SLACK Incorporated

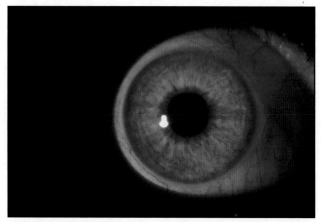

Figure 1-1. Diffuse illumination. A broad beam is used to obtain an overview of the anterior segment.

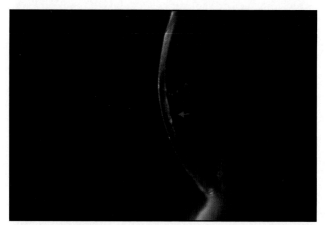

Figure 1-2. Slit illumination. A thin beam is used to visualize a section of the cornea, which gives information regarding the corneal thickness and the layer in which any abnormalities may be. The arrow indicates an area of Descemet's detachment.

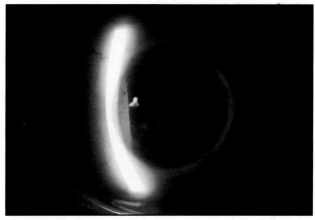

Figure 1-3. Sclerotic scatter. Central corneal scarring is visualized when light is shined at the limbus.

Sclerotic Scatter. Shine the light beam at the limbus: The light will scatter off the sclera and, because of the internal reflection of the cornea, the cornea will be dimly illuminated highlighting edema or opacities (Figure 1-3).

Retroillumination. Shine the light through the edge of the pupil: The light will reflect off the retina, giving a red reflex that will transilluminate any iris defects and highlight lens or cornea opacities (see Figures 10-8 and 10-9).

CORNEAL STAINING

Fluorescein

Fluorescein is a nontoxic, water-soluble dye that has several uses in the slit-lamp examination. It is best observed with the cobalt blue filter.

- Used for applanation tonometer testing.

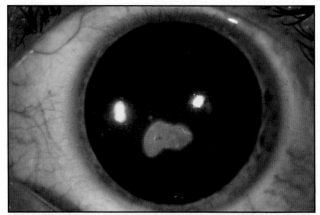

Figure 1-4. Fluorescein staining. A paracentral corneal epithelial defect is highlighted with fluorescein stain.

- Stains denuded or missing epithelial cells and is most helpful in showing epithelial defects or punctate staining in dry eye disease (Figure 1-4).
- Used to assess tear break-up time in dry eye disease—count the seconds after a blink to when a dry spot appears on the cornea.

Rose Bengal

Stains devitalized epithelial cells that have lost their mucin covering; it is more sensitive for testing conjunctiva (Figure 1-5). Rose bengal classically stains the devitalized epithelial cells at the border of a dendritic lesion in herpetic epithelial keratitis (see Figure 5-6).

Lissamine Green

Similar staining characteristics to rose bengal but better tolerated by patients (Figure 1-6).

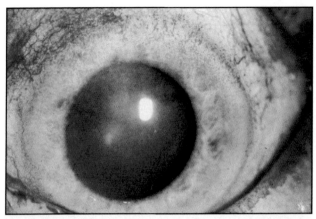

Figure 1-5. Rose bengal staining. The rose bengal stain highlights punctate epithelial erosions in the superior cornea and conjunctiva.

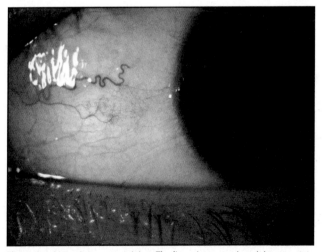

Figure 1-6. Lissamine green staining. The lissamine green is staining punctate epithelial erosions on the conjunctiva.

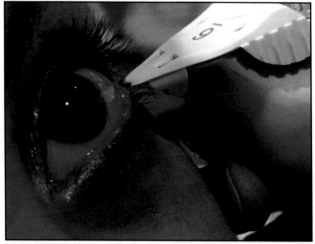

Figure 1-7. Tear osmolarity testing. A handheld device is used to sample the tear lake to determine the osmolarity.

TEAR ANALYSIS

Tear Composition Assays

Tear Osmolarity Testing. Tear osmolarity is increased in dry eye disease. A rapid assay using a handheld device that collects a small amount of tears determines the osmolarity; >300 mOsm/L is considered elevated and an intereye difference of >8 mOsm/L is considered abnormal (Figure 1-7).

Matrix Metalloproteinase 9 Testing. Matrix metalloproteinase 9 (MMP-9) is a chemical marker of inflammation in distressed epithelial cells. A rapid, single-use assay is available to test a small amount of tears for the presence of elevated MMP-9 levels (Figure 1-8).

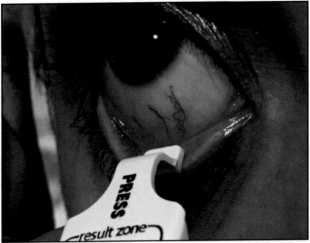

Figure 1-8. MMP-9 testing. A single-use testing cassette is used to sample the tear lake to determine the presence of MMP-9. The cassette has an indicator stripe displaying the results.

Schirmer's Testing

A test of tear production.

- Place a thin strip of filter paper in inferior cul-de-sac at the outer third of the lower eyelid and measure the amount of wetting after 5 minutes (Figure 1-9).
- Typically performed after an anesthetic drop is placed.
- < 5 mm abnormal; 5 mm to 10 mm equivocal; > 10 mm normal tear production.

OTHER CORNEAL TESTING

Corneal Pachymetry

Determines corneal thickness in microns (μm).

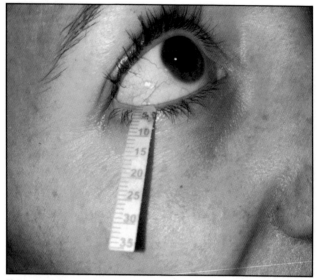

Figure 1-9. Schirmer's testing. A testing strip is placed into the fornix after topical anesthesia and read after 5 minutes.

- Average corneal thickness is 545 μm.
- Useful for monitoring endothelial cell function/corneal edema.
- Pretesting for laser vision correction.

Corneal Sensation

Corneal sensation is mediated by the ophthalmic branch of cranial nerve V. Methods for testing corneal sensation can be qualitative or quantitative. A qualitative method is to release fine strands of cotton from a cotton-tipped applicator, gently touch the corneal surface with the cotton strands, and grade the objective and subjective responses of the patient. A quantitative method is to use the Cochet-Bonnet esthesiometer, which involves extending an adjustable length of nylon filament (between 0 cm and

6 cm) toward the cornea, and assessing the longest length that produces a greater than 50% response rate. Patients with normal corneal sensation typically measure 4.5 cm or greater with the Cochet-Bonnet esthesiometer, and lengths shorter than 4.5 cm are indicative of decreased corneal sensation.

Corneal Cultures

In the case of presumed infectious keratitis, it is advised to collect cultures to identify the causative agent in cases that involve the central cornea, are larger than 2 mm, involve the deep stroma, or if you suspect an unusual pathogen.

- Collecting cultures is performed by scraping the lesion with a sterile spatula, blade, or swab. Take the specimen from the periphery of the ulcer as the center is usual necrotic, nonviable tissue.
- Inoculate plates and slides with a sterile spatula, blade or calcium alginate swab dipped in thioglycolate broth. Streak multiple "C" shapes across the plate (Figure 1-10). Slides may be stored in a nonsterile manner, and the sampling instrument (spatula, blade, or swab) should therefore be replaced with a sterile sampling instrument after coming in contact with a slide.
- Send 2 slides: 1 for Gram stain and 1 for fungal stain.
- Viral: Use Dacron swab (not cotton-tip or calcium alginate swab) and pink viral media for herpes simplex virus polymerase chain reaction.
- Blood agar is used for aerobic bacteria.
- Chocolate agar is used for *Neisseria gonorrheae* and *Haemophilus*.
- Sabouraud agar or potato dextrose is used for fungus.
- Thioglycolate broth is used for anaerobic bacteria.
- Löwenstein-Jensen is used for mycobacteria.

Depending on your clinical suspicion, you can also evaluate for acanthamoeba with a smear or attempt to culture it on nonnutrient agar with *Escherichia coli* overlay.

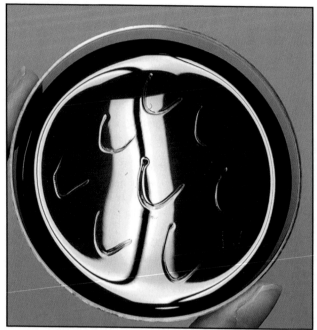

Figure 1-10. Corneal cultures. A corneal infiltrate is sampled and smeared onto a blood agar plate in multiple "C" shapes.

Take care not to contaminate your specimens: Wear gloves, do not touch the spatula to the eyelids or skin, and use a new sterile spatula for each specimen.

BIBLIOGRAPHY

1.   Weisenthal RW. *2013-2014 Basic and Clinical Science Course, Section 8: External Disease and Cornea.* San Francisco, CA: American Academy of Ophthalmology; 2014.

2

Corneal and Anterior Segment Imaging

MEASUREMENT OF CORNEAL CURVATURE

Keratometry

Keratometry measures the curvature of the central cornea, from which the power of a cornea in diopters can be estimated.[1]

Keratometry is used to measure regular astigmatism, for contact lens fitting, and in intraocular lens calculations for cataract surgery.

Typical keratometry methods compute the corneal radius of curvature by measuring the height of mire reflections off the corneal surface, which is treated as a convex mirror.

Keratometry works well for most normal corneas but the accuracy of corneal power obtained by keratometry will be limited in eyes with keratoconus and those that have undergone refractive surgery.

Kim T, Daluvoy MB.
The Pocket Guide to Cornea (pp 11-20).
© 2019 SLACK Incorporated.

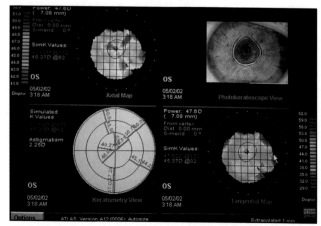

Figure 2-1. Corneal topography. This scan from a Zeiss Atlas device shows axial curvature, Placido disc images, simulated keratometry, and tangential curvature.

Corneal Topography

Corneal topography is a noninvasive imaging modality that can be used to generate maps of the anterior surface of the cornea.[2-4]

Corneal topography is widely used to evaluate patients for refractive surgery, diagnose and monitor corneal ectasia, understand the effects of neoplasms and pterygia on corneal curvature, and evaluate corneal shape after penetrating keratoplasty (PKP).

The classical form of topography is based on the Placido disc, introduced in 1880 by Antonio Placido and consisting of a series of concentric rings or mires. The later development of algorithms for the automatic detection of the mires from images allowed for the computation of color-coded maps of corneal shape and power.

The most commonly used map in routine clinical evaluation is the axial curvature map (Figure 2-1), which relates corneal power to corneal shape. On this map, normal eyes typically have smooth power contours, and right and left eyes tend to be mirror images of each other. While the axial curvature map may underestimate peripheral corneal power, its emphasis on corneal shape makes it particularly useful in the identification of patients at risk for corneal ectasia.

In addition to the axial curvature map, refractive power maps, instantaneous curvature maps, difference maps, and elevation maps can be computed.

Slit-Scanning Corneal Tomography

Slit-scanning corneal tomography uses light scattered both from the anterior and posterior corneal surfaces when illuminated with a slit beam to generate pachymetry maps and elevation maps of the anterior and posterior corneal surfaces, providing a 3-dimensional representation of the cornea.[5-7]

Elevation maps can be used in the identification of keratoconus, as posterior corneal elevation may be one of the initial changes (Figure 2-2A showing regular astigmatism, Figure 2-2B with keratoconus). Like topography, these images are used to evaluate patients for refractive surgery, diagnose and monitor corneal ectasia, understand the effects of neoplasms and pterygia on corneal curvature, and evaluate corneal shape after PKP.

Anterior Segment Optical Coherence Tomography

Anterior segment optical coherence tomography (ASOCT) uses interferometry to generate cross-sectional images of the anterior segment (Figure 2 3).[8-10]

ASOCT provides information regarding corneal curvature, thickness, and opacities.

Segmentation of optical coherence tomography (OCT) images can allow for the generation of curvature and pachymetry maps, which can be of use in the evaluation of corneal ectasia.

For patients with corneal opacities, OCT can be used to identify the depth of the opacity, which can in turn aid in determining whether surgical intervention is appropriate and, if so, which type.

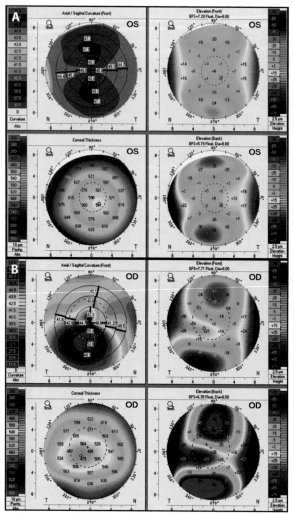

Figure 2-2. Corneal tomography. (A) This shows regular corneal astigmatism with normal corneal thickness. (B) This shows inferior steepening and corneal thinning consistent with keratoconus.

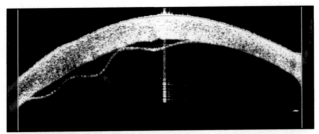

Figure 2-3. ASOCT. A cross-sectional image of the cornea demonstrates a Descemet detachment (red arrow).

ASOCT can also be used to evaluate surgically altered corneas (particularly after lamellar keratoplasty) because of its excellent depth resolution (3 μm to 5 μm with modern systems). In particular, ASOCT is helpful in the determination of Descemet stripping endothelial keratoplasty and Descemet membrane endothelial keratoplasty graft attachment after endothelial keratoplasty, as edematous stroma can limit the examiner's view of the posterior cornea and anterior chamber.

High-resolution ASOCT systems are also used for the evaluation and differentiation of neoplasms of the ocular surface, including ocular surface squamous neoplasia, lymphoma, and melanoma.

Ultrasound Biomicroscopy

Ultrasound biomicroscopy (UBM) uses high-frequency ultrasound (25 MHz to 100 MHz) to obtain cross-sectional images of the anterior segment and ocular adnexa (Figure 2-4).[11-13]

The high frequency utilized by UBM offers higher axial resolution than traditional ultrasound (20 μm to 40 μm for UBM vs 50 μm to 150 μm for traditional ultrasound) at the expense of limited penetration into tissues (focal range typically 1 mm to 5 mm with UBM vs 15 mm to 35 mm for traditional ultrasound).

UBM is typically performed with the use of a fluid-coupling agent between the eye and the scanning ultrasound probe.

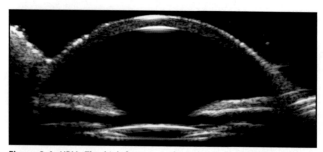

Figure 2-4. UBM. The high-frequency ultrasound image captures a normal anterior segment.

While the resolution of UBM is lower than that of advanced commercial ASOCT systems (3 μm to 5 μm), UBM offers additional flexibility in imaging. In particular, because of its use of sound, UBM is able to image opaque tissues, including eyelids, sclera, and pathologically altered corneas. It can additionally be used to assess anterior segment tumors, the state of the lens, iris configuration, and the state of the iridocorneal angle. Furthermore, visualization of the internal structures of the anterior segment in an eye with an opaque cornea can be essential to surgical planning, and cannot be achieved with optical imaging systems.

Specular Microscopy

Specular microscopy is a rapid, noncontact imaging modality that is typically used to evaluate the corneal endothelium and Descemet membrane.[14,15]

Specular microscopy relies on specular (or mirror-like) reflection at an optical interface. In clinical practice, the interface of interest is typically the corneal endothelial-aqueous interface. Observation of light reflected from this interface provides an image of the corneal endothelial cells. Systematic capture of multiple images of the corneal endothelium, including central,

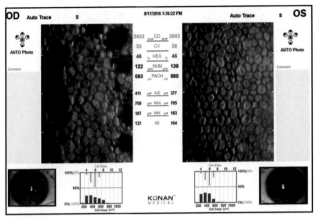

Figure 2-5. Specular microscopy. The readout gives information about endothelial cell density, volume, and morphology. The round, dark, "punched-out" areas on the image represent guttae.

midperipheral, and peripheral endothelium, can allow for qualitative and quantitative analysis of the endothelium.

The size, shape, and density of the corneal endothelial cells are analyzed (Figure 2-5).

Quantitative analysis of the endothelial cells allows for monitoring of endothelial disease (eg, Fuchs' endothelial dystrophy or pseudophakic bullous keratopathy) as well as tracking of outcomes after surgical intervention for endothelial disease.

Confocal Microscopy

Confocal microscopy is used to study the specific cell layers of the cornea even in cases of scarring or edema.[16-19]

Confocal microscopy refers to the use of a point source (light) focused at a given location within a tissue, and a point detector focused at the same location within the tissue. The reduction of the light source size allows for elimination of contributions from neighboring regions within the tissue of interest, thereby increasing potential resolution. To generate an image with a useful field

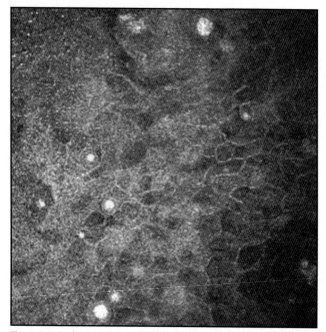

Figure 2-6. Confocal microscopy. Multiple double-walled cysts can be visualized in this patient with acanthamoeba keratitis.

of view, the location of the point of interest is scanned within a given plane and then integrated into a single image. Images can be generated at multiple depths to create a "stack" of images spanning epithelium to endothelium.

Confocal microscopy offers resolution of 1 μm to 2 μm transversely and 4 μm axially. This level of detail allows one to examine epithelial cells, keratocytes, inflammatory cells, the subbasal nerve plexus, and endothelial cells.

Confocal microscopy is most commonly used for evaluation of infectious keratitis (especially parasitic [Figure 2-6] and fungal forms), corneal inflammatory disease, wound healing after refractive surgery, and corneal nerve density as an indicator of corneal disease and systemic neuropathies.

Meibomian Gland Imaging

Meibomian gland imaging is used to evaluate for atrophy or dropout of Meibomian glands and their ducts (see Figure 3-3).

Most modern forms of Meibomian gland imaging (meibography) involve illumination of the everted eyelid with an infrared light source and image capture with an infrared camera.

While no single standard scale for grading Meibomian gland images exists, most published grading scales assess the proportion of Meibomian gland acini visible and the presence or absence of Meibomian gland ducts.

Meibography can be used as a tool to assess the severity of the evaporative component of dry eye.

REFERENCES

1. Emsley H. Keratometry. In: *Visual Optics*. London, England: Hatton Press Ltd; 1946:298-324.

2. Bogan SJ, Waring GO III, Ibrahim O, Drews C, Curtis L. Classification of normal corneal topography based on computer-assisted video-keratography. *Arch Ophthalmol*. 1990;108(7):945-949. doi:10.1001/archopht.1990.01070090047037.

3. Dingeldein SA, Klyce SD, Wilson SE. Quantitative descriptors of corneal shape derived from computer-assisted analysis of photokeratographs. *Refract Corneal Surg*. 5(6):372-378. doi:10.3928/1081-597X-19891101-06.

4. Klyce SD. Computer-assisted corneal topography. High-resolution graphic presentation and analysis of keratoscopy. *Invest Ophthalmol Vis Sci*. 1984;25(12):1426-1435.

5. de Sanctis U, Loiacono C, Richiardi L, Turco D, Mutani B, Grignolo FM. Sensitivity and specificity of posterior corneal elevation measured by Pentacam in discriminating keratoconus/subclinical keratoconus. *Ophthalmology*. 2008;115(9):1534-1539. doi:10.1016/j.ophtha.2008.02.020.

6. Tanabe T, Oshika T, Tomidokoro A, et al. Standardized color-coded scales for anterior and posterior elevation maps of scanning slit corneal topography. *Ophthalmology*. 2002;109(7):1298-1302. doi:10.1016/S0161-6420(02)01030-8.

7. Yaylali V, Kaufman SC, Thompson HW. Corneal thickness measurements with the Orbscan Topography System and ultrasonic pachymetry. *J Cataract Refract Surg.* 1997;23(9):1345-1350. doi:10.1016/S0886-3350(97)80113-7.

8. Huang D, Swanson EA, Lin CP, et al. Optical coherence tomography. *Science.* 1991;254(5035):1178-1181. doi:10.1126/science.1957169.

9. Izatt JA, Hee MR, Swanson EA, et al. Micrometer-scale resolution imaging of the anterior eye in vivo with optical coherence tomography. *Arch Ophthalmol.* 1994;112(12):1584-1589. doi:10.1001/archopht.1994.01090240090031.

10. Khurana RN, Li Y, Tang M, Lai MM, Huang D. High-speed optical coherence tomography of corneal opacities. *Ophthalmology.* 2007;114(7):1278-1285. doi:10.1016/j.ophtha.2006.10.033.

11. Foster FS, Pavlin CJ, Harasiewicz KA, Christopher DA, Turnbull DH. Advances in ultrasound biomicroscopy. *Ultrasound Med Biol.* 2000;26(1):1-27. doi:10.1016/S0301-5629(99)00096-4.

12. Pavlin CJ, Harasiewicz K, Sherar MD, Foster FS. Clinical use of ultrasound biomicroscopy. *Ophthalmology.* 1991;98(3):287-295. doi:10.1016/S0161-6420(91)32298-X.

13. Pavlin CJ, Sherar MD, Foster FS. Subsurface ultrasound microscopic imaging of the intact eye. *Ophthalmology.* 1990;97(2):244-250. doi:10.1016/S0161-6420(90)32598-8.

14. Laing RA, Leibowitz HM, Oak SS, Chang R, Berrospi AR, Theodore J. Endothelial mosaic in Fuchs' dystrophy. A qualitative evaluation with the specular microscope. *Arch Ophthalmol.* 1981;99(1):80-83. doi:10.1001/archopht.1981.03930010082007.

15. Laing RA, Sandstrom MM, Leibowitz HM. In vivo photomicrography of the corneal endothelium. *Arch Ophthalmol.* 1975;93(2):143-145. doi:10.1001/archopht.1975.01010020149013.

16. Auran JD, Starr MB, Koester CJ, La Bombardi VJ. In vivo scanning slit confocal microscopy of Acanthamoeba keratitis. *Cornea.* 1994;13(2):183-185.

17. Lukosz W. Optical systems with resolving powers exceeding the classical limit. *J Opt Soc Am.* 1966;56(11):1463-1471. doi:10.1364/JOSA.56.001463.

18. Minsky M. Memoir on inventing the confocal scanning microscope. *Scanning J.* 1988;10:128-138. doi:10.1002/sca.4950100403.

19. Wilson T. Confocal light microscopy. *Ann NY Acad Sci.* 1986;483:416-427. doi:10.1111/j.1749-6632.1986.tb34551.x.

3

Dry Eye Disease

AQUEOUS TEAR DEFICIENCY

Inflammation of the lacrimal gland causes reduced tear production and release of inflammatory mediators onto the ocular surface.

Signs and Symptoms. Burning, blurry vision, symptoms worsening at the end of the day, decreased tear meniscus (<0.3 mm), punctate epithelial erosions/superficial punctate keratopathy (Figure 3-1), and filaments or keratinization in severe disease.

Exams and Tests. Slit-lamp examination with fluorescein, lissamine green, or rose bengal staining; Schirmer's testing (<15 mm in 5 minutes abnormal without topical anesthetic, <5 mm in 5 minutes with anesthetic), tear osmolarity (normal <302 mOsm/L; mild/moderate dry eye disease >315 mOsm/L; severe dry eye disease >336 mOsm/L), positive matrix metalloproteinase 9 (MMP-9) assay, and consider systemic evaluation for Sjögren's syndrome.

Treatment. Artificial tears, gel, or ointment (especially preservative-free formulations), topical cyclosporine 0.5%, lifitegrast (Xiidra,

Kim T, Daluvoy MB.
The Pocket Guide to Cornea (pp 21-25).
© 2019 SLACK Incorporated.

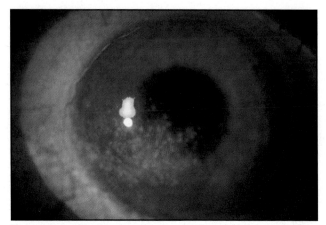

Figure 3-1. Superficial punctate keratopathy. Fluorescein staining highlights coarse punctate epithelial erosions.

Shire), autologous serum drops, punctal occlusion (plugs for temporary effect, cautery for permanent result), moisture chamber goggles, omega-3 fatty acid supplementation, smoking cessation, discontinuation of drops containing preservatives, serum tears, scleral contact lenses, or tarsorrhaphy in advanced cases.

EVAPORATIVE DRY EYE

Meibomian gland dysfunction leads to poor lipid quality, which causes tear film instability, rapid evaporation of tears, and tear hyperosmolarity. Meibomian gland dysfunction can be secondary to conditions affecting the eyelids, such as ocular rosacea, atopic keratoconjunctivitis, and mucous membrane pemphigoid.

Signs and Symptoms. Burning, blurry vision, worsening of symptoms in the morning, foam or debris in tear film, telangiectatic vessels at eyelid margin, plugging of Meibomian gland orifices (Figure 3-2), viscous Meibomian gland secretions, and Meibomian gland atrophy.

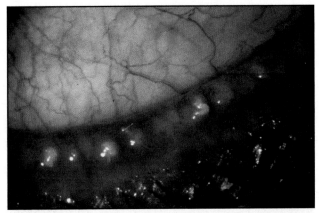

Figure 3-2. Meibomian gland dysfunction. External photograph shows multiple inspissated Meibomian glands and eyelid margin telangiectasias.

Exams and Tests. Tear break-up time (<10 seconds abnormal), tear osmolarity (>300 mOsm abnormal), MMP-9 assay, and dynamic Meibomian gland imaging (Figure 3-3).

Treatment. Artificial tears, gel, or ointment, warm compresses, eyelid hygiene (with commercially prepared eyelid scrubs, baby shampoo, or diluted tea tree oil shampoo), doxycycline, Meibomian gland expression (manually or with devices such as LipiFlow, TearScience), and intense pulsed light (for patients with ocular rosacea).

FILAMENTARY KERATITIS

Collection of devitalized epithelial cells attached to a mucous core usually seen in severe dry eye.

Signs and Symptoms. Pain, foreign body sensation, photophobia, dryness, and filaments attached to corneal surface.

Exams and Tests. Slit-lamp examination with fluorescein staining (will stain filaments; Figure 3-4).

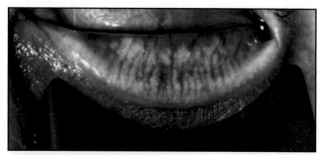

Figure 3-3. Meibography. The lower eyelid is everted, and the image captures the normal-appearing linear Meibomian glands.

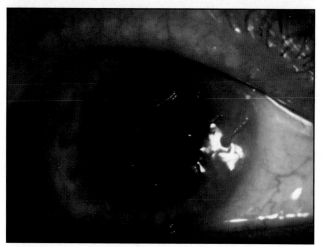

Figure 3-4. Filamentary keratitis. Multiple strands of devitalized epithelial cells are attached to mucous adherent to the cornea.

Treatment. Debridement of filaments with forceps, acetylcysteine 10% drops, aggressive lubrication or punctal occlusion, bandage contact lenses, and correction of eyelid abnormalities that may be contributing to surface disease.

BIBLIOGRAPHY

1. Nelson JD, Craig JP, Akpek EK, et al. TFOS International Dry Eye Workshop (DEWS II). *Ocul Surf.* 2017;15(3):269-275. doi:10.1016/j.jtos.2017.05.005.
2. Holland E, Luchs J, Karpecki PM, et al. Lifitegrast for the treatment of dry eye disease: results of a phase III, randomized, double-masked, placebo-controlled trial (OPUS-3). *Ophthalmology.* 2017;124(1):53-60. doi:10.1016/j.ophtha.2016.09.025.

4

Eyelid Conditions Affecting the Ocular Surface

BLEPHARITIS

An inflammation of the eyelid margin, blepharitis is typically classified as anterior or posterior, although there is much overlap. Anterior blepharitis affects the eyelid skin, eyelashes, and follicles while posterior blepharitis affects the Meibomian glands and orifices and is often referred to as Meibomian gland dysfunction.

Signs and Symptoms. Swelling, thickening, scaling, crusting, and telangiectasia of eyelid margins, thick and turbid secretions from Meibomian glands, plugged Meibomian glands, conjunctival injection, irritation, itching, burning, and blurred vision.

Exams and Tests. External and slit-lamp examination with careful attention to eyelid margin and expression of Meibomian glands. Test for rapid tear break-up time, tear film assays, and Meibomian gland imaging (in vivo visualization of the morphology of the Meibomian glands. See Figure 3-3).

Treatment. Eyelid hygiene consists of gentle eyelid scrubs with a mild soap and warm water BID. Warm compresses for 10 to 15 minutes

Kim T, Daluvoy MB.
The Pocket Guide to Cornea (pp 27-33).
© 2019 SLACK Incorporated.

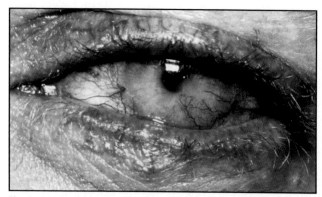

Figure 4-1. Ocular rosacea. An advanced case of ocular rosacea depicting eyelid erythema and telangiectasias, conjunctival injection, and corneal neovascularization.

BID, lubrication, omega-3 supplements, topical antibiotic drops and ointments, topical steroids as needed, oral tetracyclines (doxycycline 100 mg BID then taper). In-office treatments, such as intense pulsed light or thermal pulsation (LipiFlow, TearScience), may be offered.

OCULAR ROSACEA

Rosacea is an inflammatory condition affecting the skin, chest, and eyes. It leads to dysfunction of the cutaneous sebaceous glands and is a major cause of Meibomian gland dysfunction.

Signs and Symptoms. Redness, burning, chronic eye irritation, conjunctival injection, peripheral corneal neovascularization, eyelid margin telangiectasia, chalazia, skin pustules, and rhinophyma. Symptoms are more common in females but can be more severe in men and can also be seen in children (Figure 4-1).

Exams and Tests. See Blepharitis.

Treatment. See Blepharitis. Metronidazole can be used on the facial lesions.

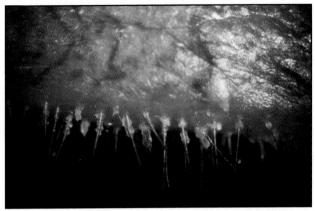

Figure 4-2. Ocular blepharitis. Scurf is visualized at the base of the eyelashes.

SEBORRHEIC BLEPHARITIS

Inflammation of the anterior eyelid margin characterized by flaking and greasy skin on the scalp, retroauricular area, and nasalobial folds.

Signs and Symptoms. Burning, irritation, blurred vision, characterized by mild eyelid redness and crusting and scaling around the eyelashes (Figure 4-2).

Exams and Tests. See Blepharitis.

Treatment. See Blepharitis.

STAPHYLOCOCCAL BLEPHARITIS

Chronic blepharitis caused by colonization with staphylococci (aureus and coagulase negative). By various mechanisms these bacteria disrupt the normal lipid tear film layer and induce inflammation.

Signs and Symptoms. Redness, burning, blurred vision, chronic irritation, misdirected or missing eyelashes. Can be associated with corneal changes such as neovascularization and phlyctenules.

Exams and Tests. See Blepharitis.

Treatment. See Blepharitis.

DEMODEX INFESTATION

Demodex infestation refers to blepharitis caused by infestation of Demodex mites.

Signs and Symptoms. Characteristic cylindrical sleeves around the eyelashes and other typical signs of blepharitis. Demodex can be present in asymptomatic individuals.

Exams and Tests. Slit-lamp examination. An individual eyelash can be pulled and inspected microscopically to confirm the diagnosis.

Treatment. In addition to traditional blepharitis treatment, tea tree oil eyelid scrubs can be effective.

CHALAZION

A localized granulomatous reaction in the setting of dysfunction of the Meibomian or Zeis glands.

Signs and Symptoms. An eyelid nodule associated with surrounding redness (Figure 4-3). Typically painless, it can cause visual changes due to induced astigmatism.

Exams and Tests. Slit-lamp examination.

Treatment. Warm compresses and steroid/antibiotic ointment. Sometimes incision and drainage is required.

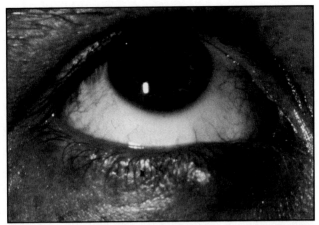

Figure 4-3. Chalazion. A blockage of the Meibomian gland orifice causes a back-up of oil.

HORDEOLUM

Localized inflammation and/or infection of an eyelash follicle or Meibomian gland of the eyelid.

Signs and Symptoms. Red, tender eyelid nodule. Presentation is typically more acute than chalazia.

Exams and Tests. Slit-lamp examination.

Treatment. See Chalazion.

FLOPPY EYELID SYNDROME

Characterized by lax upper tarsus that everts with minimal pressure causing chronic irritation to the exposed bulbar and palpebral conjunctiva, especially while sleeping.

Signs and Symptoms. Typically, in obese patients, floppy eyelid syndrome is associated with sleep apnea. Eyelids can be easily

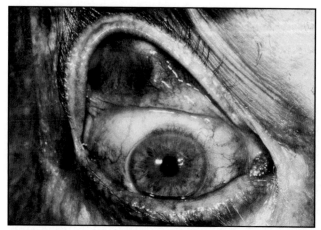

Figure 4-4. Floppy eyelid syndrome. The upper eyelid can be easily and fully everted with minimal effort. The tarsal conjunctiva demonstrates a papillary reaction.

everted, pulled away from the globe (Figure 4-4), with a long snap back time. Fine papillary response on palpebral surface, mucous discharge, corneal punctate epithelial erosions (PEEs), and neovascularization.

Exams and Tests. External and slit-lamp examinations.

Treatment. Recommend a sleep study evaluation for sleep apnea, sleeping with shields or other eye protection, surgical correction of eyelid laxity, nighttime lubrication, and treatment of dry eye symptoms.

EXPOSURE KERATOPATHY

Corneal findings due to improper closure of the eyelids (lagophthalmos, Figure 4-5). There are many etiologies: poor blink, Parkinson disease, cranial nerve VII palsy, ectropion, thyroid eye disease, conjunctival scarring, and aggressive blepharoplasty.

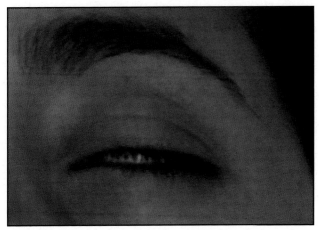

Figure 4-5. Lagophthalmos. Incomplete eyelid closure can lead to exposure keratopathy.

Signs and Symptoms. Redness, irritation, photophobia, foreign body sensation, and dense PEEs in exposed area; be suspicious of poor nighttime closure when PEEs are dense inferiorly.

Exams and Tests. External and slit-lamp examination. Ask family members about exposure while sleeping.

Treatment. Aggressive lubrication, nighttime ointment or gels, tape tarsorrhaphy, surgical tarsorrhaphy, surgery to repair eyelid abnormality, and gold-weight insertion in upper eyelid.

BIBLIOGRAPHY

1.   Pflugfelder SC, Karpecki PM, Perez VL. Treatment of blepharitis: recent clinical trials. *Ocul Surf.* 2014;12(4):273-284. doi:10.1016/j.jtos.2014.05.005.

5

Infectious Conditions

CONJUNCTIVA

Bacterial Conjunctivitis

Gonococcal. Infection of the conjunctiva caused by *Neisseria gonorrhoeae*, usually sexually transmitted from direct or indirect contact (Table 5-1).

Signs and Symptoms. Rapid onset and progression of purulent discharge (Figure 5-1), severe hyperemia, chemosis, eyelid edema, preauricular lymphadenopathy, and conjunctival membranes. Corneal infiltrate and melting can occur if untreated. Patients may have associated urethritis, vaginitis, or cervicitis.

Exams and Tests. Conjunctival swab and Gram stain to identify intracellular Gram-negative diplococci; culture on chocolate agar, blood agar, and Thayer-Martin media.

Treatment. Irrigate conjunctival sac at least QID to remove inflammatory mediators and debris. If there is no corneal involvement, it can be treated with a single dose of 1 g ceftriaxone

Kim T, Daluvoy MB.
The Pocket Guide to Cornea (pp 35-50).
© 2019 SLACK Incorporated.

Table 5-1. Differential Diagnosis for Neonatal Conjunctivitis

Within 24 to 48 hours after birth	Chemical (usually related to instillation of silver nitrate)
Within 2 to 5 days after birth	Gonorrheal
Within 6 to 14 days after birth	Chlamydial
	Herpes simplex virus

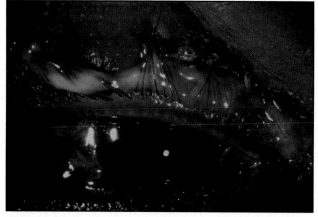

Figure 5-1. Gonococcal conjunctivitis. There is copious purulent discharge and severe hyperemia with a hyperacute onset.

intramuscularly (IM). If there is corneal involvement, treat with 1 g ceftriaxone intravenously (IV) BID for 3 days. Alternatives include single dose of spectinomycin 2 g IM or ciprofloxacin 500 mg PO BID for 5 days. Topical adjunctive therapy includes antibiotic ointment (erythromycin, bacitracin, or gentamicin) or ciprofloxacin drops if there is corneal involvement. Also consider treating for chlamydia given high incidence of co-occurrence.

Chlamydial-Trachoma. Infection caused by *Chlamydia trachomatis* serotypes A through C, mostly in areas of poor hygiene and sanitation. Transmission occurs eye to eye but can also occur through flies.

Signs and Symptoms. Foreign body sensation, mucopurulent discharge, conjunctival follicular reaction, scarring of the superior tarsus (Arlt line), round scarring of limbal follicles (Herbert pits), epithelial keratitis, stromal infiltrates, and fibrovascular pannus especially superiorly. Late findings include trichiasis, entropion, and corneal scarring.

Exams and Tests. Giemsa stain, direct fluorescent antibody staining, chlamydial culture, and polymerase chain reaction (PCR) probes.

Treatment. Systemic treatment with a single dose of 1 g azithromycin PO, doxycycline 100 mg PO BID for 2 weeks, tetracycline 250 mg PO QID for 2 weeks, or erythromycin 500 mg PO QID for 2 weeks. Topical therapy is recommended with tetracycline 1%, erythromycin, or sulfacetamide ointment BID-QID for 1 to 2 months. Address trichiasis to prevent corneal scarring. Improve hygiene to prevent reinfection.

Chlamydial-Inclusion Conjunctivitis. Infection of the conjunctiva caused by *Chlamydia trachomatis* serotypes D through K, transmitted sexually or through direct or indirect contact.

Signs and Symptoms. Foreign body sensation, mucopurulent discharge over 3 to 4 weeks, conjunctival follicles, preauricular lymphadenopathy, corneal epithelial keratitis, and micropannus superiorly. Patients may have associated urethritis, vaginitis, or cervicitis.

Exams and Tests. Giemsa stain, direct fluorescent antibody staining, chlamydial culture, and PCR probes.

Treatment. Single dose of 1 g azithromycin PO, doxycycline 100 mg PO BID for 7 days, tetracycline 250 mg PO QID for 7 days, or erythromycin 500 mg PO QID for 7 days. Also consider treating for gonorrhea given high incidence of co-occurrence.

Other Bacterial Conjunctivitis (non-Gonococcal) Infection of the conjunctiva usually caused by direct contact with infected

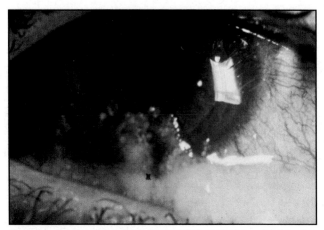

Figure 5-2. Bacterial conjunctivitis. Purulent discharge is observed, but to a less severe degree and with a slower onset than gonococcal conjunctivitis.

secretions or adjacent spread from nasal or sinus mucosa. Common organisms include *Staphylococcus aureus*, *Haemophilus influenzae*, and *Streptococcus pneumoniae*.

Signs and Symptoms. Redness, conjunctival papillae, and purulent discharge (Figure 5-2). Conjunctival membranes may be seen with severe *S. pneumoniae* infections. Preauricular lymphadenopathy is usually absent.

Exams and Tests. Consider conjunctival swab for Gram stain and culture if there is suspicion for hyperacute gonococcal conjunctivitis, in immunocompromised patients, or if a patient has recurrent or recalcitrant symptoms.

Treatment. Most cases are self-limited and self-resolve after one week. Topical treatments include broad-spectrum agents such as polymyxin B/trimethoprim, gentamicin, tobramycin, or fluoroquinolone drops or ointment QID for one week. If *H. influenzae*, systemic therapy with amoxicillin/clavulanate is recommended to treat extraocular manifestations.

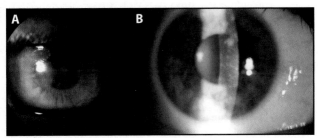

Figure 5-3. Viral conjunctivitis. (A) Diffuse illumination showing multiple discrete, round opacities representing subepithelial infiltrates. (B) Slit-beam photograph showing subepithelial infiltrates.

Viral Conjunctivitis

Highly contagious infection of the conjunctiva usually caused by adenovirus. Epidemic keratoconjunctivitis (EKC) is caused by serotypes 8, 19, 37, or subgroup D.

Signs and Symptoms. Conjunctival injection, itching, watery discharge, conjunctival follicles, and petechial conjunctival hemorrhages. EKC can lead to membranes or pseudomembranes and preauricular lymphadenopathy, and corneal subepithelial infiltrates can occur days to weeks after onset (Figure 5-3).

Exams and Tests. Clinical diagnosis is preferred. No laboratory workup is indicated unless severe or chronic. Fast-acting tear assays are available to test for adenovirus but rarely used.

Treatment. Viral conjunctivitis is self-limited in most cases but is highly contagious, so emphasize hand hygiene. Symptoms can be managed with artificial tears and cool compresses. Itching can be managed with topical antihistamines. If membranes or pseudomembranes are present, remove with forceps and apply topical corticosteroids QID. If visually significant corneal subepithelial infiltrates are present, treat with slow taper of low-potency topical steroids or topical cyclosporine 0.5%.

Parinaud Oculoglandular Syndrome

Granulomatous conjunctivitis and regional lymphadenopathy most commonly caused by *Bartonella henselae* through infected kittens or infected fleas (Cat Scratch disease). Other causes include tularemia, tuberculosis, sporotrichosis, syphilis, and coccidioidomycosis.

Signs and Symptoms. Redness, foreign body sensation, unilateral granulomatous lesions on the conjunctiva or fornix, ipsilateral preauricular, submandibular, or cervical lymphadenopathy. Systemic symptoms such as fever, headache, and malaise may be present.

Exams and Tests. Indirect fluorescent antibody testing or enzyme immunoassay for *B. henselae*. Depending on other systemic symptoms, consider workup for other causative organisms.

Treatment. Systemic therapy should be based on specific cause. Possible agents include azithromycin, erythromycin, doxycycline, rifampin, trimethoprim-sulfamethoxazole, and fluoroquinolones.

CORNEAL INFECTIONS

Bacterial Keratitis

Bacterial infection of the cornea most commonly caused by *Staphylococcus aureus*, *Staphylococcus epidermidis*, *Streptococcus species*, *Pseudomonas aeruginosa* (especially in contact lens wearers), *Enterobacter*, *Haemophilus*, and *Moraxella*.

Signs and Symptoms. Pain, photophobia, redness, decreased vision, single white stromal infiltrate usually with overlying epithelial defect, well-defined borders, and corneal edema. Pseudomonas ulcers may cause suppurative inflammation with endothelial plaque and hypopyon (Figure 5-4).

Exam and Tests. Slit-lamp examination with fluorescein staining, corneal scraping and cultures if >2 mm or central. Consider

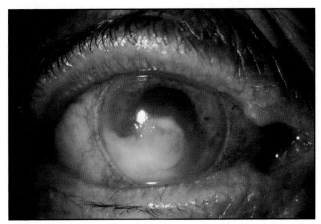

Figure 5-4. Pseudomonas keratitis. A round corneal infiltrate is surrounded by suppurative inflammation and an endothelial plaque.

corneal biopsy if unresponsive to therapy with recurrent negative cultures.

Treatment. Empiric therapy with broad-spectrum topical antibiotics every 30 to 60 minutes initially: fluoroquinolone for small ulcers, fortified tobramycin 14 mg/mL, fortified ceftazidime 50 mg/mL, or fortified cefazolin 50 mg/mL for larger ulcers. If suspicion for Gram-positive cocci, add fortified vancomycin 25 mg/mL. Consider subconjunctival antibiotics if poor compliance. Discontinue contact lens wear. Cycloplegic can be used for comfort. Taper antibiotic choice and frequency according to culture results and clinical response. Use of topical corticosteroids is controversial in the absence of a culture-proven organism. For ulcers with a positive bacterial culture, the Steroids for Corneal Ulcers Trial indicates there may be a small visual acuity benefit if topical steroids are started 48 hours after antibiotic initiation for certain subgroups, including patients with counting fingers or worse vision on presentation, patients with central ulcers of greater than 4 mm diameter, and non-Nocardia ulcers.

Nontuberculous Mycobacterial Keratitis

Infection of the cornea caused by mycobacteria such as *M. fortuitum* and *M. cheloni*, most commonly seen in post-LASIK patients.

Signs and Symptoms. Pain, redness, decreased vision, photophobia, delayed onset after refractive surgery, diffuse haze, and infiltrate.

Exams and Tests. Corneal scraping (may need to lift LASIK flap) and culture on Löwenstein-Jensen media, acid-fast stain.

Treatment. Fourth-generation topical fluoroquinolone, amikacin 15 mg/mL, clarithromycin 1% to 4%, or tobramycin 14 mg/mL.

Viral Keratitis

Herpes Simplex Keratitis. This relatively common infection is due to herpes simplex virus (HSV) type 1 with several different presentations. It can present as a primary infection or recurrent infection caused by reactivation of the virus, which lies latent in the sensory ganglion. Recurrent HSV can affect almost any ocular tissue, but most commonly affects the cornea.

Blepharoconjunctivitis. Most common presentation of primary infection affecting eyelids and conjunctiva.

Signs and Symptoms. Vesicular rash around eyelid, eyelid edema, conjunctival follicular reaction (Figure 5-5).

Exams and Tests. Usually clinical diagnosis, but if uncertain can consider scraping vesicle and performing cytology, enzyme-linked immunosorbent assay (ELISA), or PCR.

Treatment. Usually self-limited, but can consider topical or systemic antiviral agents (see below) to shorten course or prevent corneal involvement.

Epithelial Keratitis

Signs and Symptoms. Pain, photophobia, redness, punctate epithelial keratitis that coalesces into dendritic epithelial lesion, and terminal bulbs on dendrites (Figure 5-6).

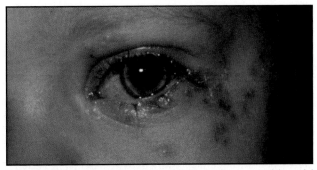

Figure 5-5. HSV blepharoconjunctivitis. A vesicular rash is seen around the eyelid with associated conjunctival injection.

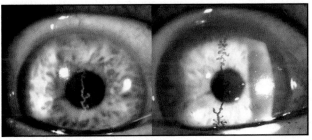

Figure 5-6. HSV epithelial keratitis. There is a dendritic lesion with terminal bulbs that stains robustly with rose bengal. (Reprinted with permission from Justin M. Roman, MD, MS.)

Exams and Tests. Corneal sensation prior to administration of topical anesthetic (often decreased sensation), slit-lamp examination with fluorescein or rose bengal staining (stains dendrites). If diagnosis is uncertain, consider corneal scraping with Dacron swab for ELISA or PCR.

Treatment. Owing to the ocular surface toxicity of topical antivirals, systemic antivirals are typically preferred (acyclovir 400 mg PO 5 times a day, valacyclovir 500 mg TID, or famciclovir 250 mg TID). Topical antivirals (ganciclovir ointment 0.15% 5 times a day or trifluridine 1% 9 times a day) can be used if renal function precludes use of systemic antivirals. Typical courses of antivirals are 7 to 14 days in duration but can be extended as needed. Topical corticosteroids are contraindicated, as their use can precipitate geographic ulceration.

Stromal Keratitis

Signs and Symptoms. Pain, photophobia, stromal haze or infiltrate, and stromal edema. Disciform keratitis presents with a discrete round area of endothelial and stromal edema with intact epithelium, keratic precipitates, and iridocyclitis. Necrotizing herpetic keratitis presents as a suppurative infiltrate resembling bacterial keratitis, epithelial defect, iridocyclitis, corneal thinning, possible hypopyon.

Exams and Tests. Corneal sensation prior to administration of topical anesthetic (often decreased sensation). If diagnosis is uncertain, consider corneal scraping with Dacron swab for ELISA or PCR.

Treatment. Topical corticosteroid (prednisolone acetate 1% every 2 hours) with slow taper, antiviral prophylaxis (acyclovir 400 mg PO BID, valacyclovir 500 mg PO daily, or famciclovir 250 mg BID) in the absence of epithelial keratitis. Prophylaxis is indicated for patients with multiple recurrences of HSV stromal keratitis and corneal scarring nearing visual axis, patients with more than one prior episode of HSV epithelial keratitis, patients with a history of HSV keratitis undergoing ocular surgery, and patients with a history of ocular HSV undergoing ocular immunosuppression.

Herpes Zoster Keratitis.

Corneal infection caused by reactivation of the varicella zoster virus (primary infection is chicken pox). The virus lies dormant in neural ganglia and reactivates later as shingles (skin involvement) or zoster ophthalmicus (ocular involvement from cranial nerve V). Typically seen in elderly or immunocompromised individuals.

Signs and Symptoms. Painful unilateral dermatomal rash (involvement of the tip of the nose predicts greater ocular involvement—Hutchinson's sign; Figure 5-7), photophobia, tearing, follicular conjunctivitis, corneal pseudodendrites (lack of terminal bulb; Figure 5-8), stromal keratitis, iridocyclitis, sectoral iris atrophy,

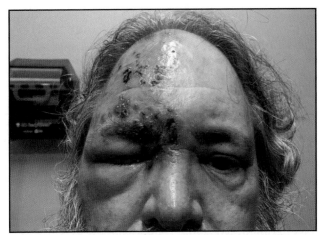

Figure 5-7. Herpes zoster ophthalmicus. A unilateral vesicular rash that has become crusted is distributed along the V1 dermatome. There is also involvement of the tip of the nose, signifying a greater chance of ocular involvement.

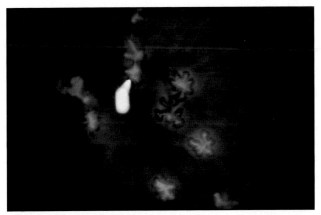

Figure 5-8. Herpes zoster keratitis. There are multiple corneal pseudodendrites (lack a terminal bulb) that stain poorly with fluorescein.

nummular corneal infiltrates, disciform keratitis, neurotrophic keratitis.

Exams and Tests. Corneal sensation testing prior to administration of topical anesthetic (often decreased sensation), slit-lamp examination with fluorescein (poor staining of pseudodendrites) and rose bengal staining (moderate staining of pseudodendrites). If young patient without known immunocompromise, test for HIV.

Treatment. Systemic antivirals (acyclovir 800 mg PO 5 times a day, valacyclovir 1 g PO TID, or famciclovir 500 mg PO TID). If immunocompromised, intravenous acyclovir 10 mg/kg TID for 7 to 10 days with subsequent transition to PO acyclovir. Add topical corticosteroid and cycloplegic if iridocyclitis or stromal keratitis present. Amytriptyline 25 mg PO TID may help prevent development of postherpetic neuralgia.

Less Common Viral Corneal Infections

Epstein-Barr Virus. Unilateral or bilateral keratitis caused by the ubiquitous Epstein-Barr virus (EBV) usually spread through saliva.

Signs and Symptoms. Foreign body sensation, redness, follicular conjunctivitis, multifocal stromal keratitis, subepithelial infiltrates, peripheral corneal vascularization.

Exams and Tests. Antiviral capsid antigen antibodies (immunoglobulin [Ig]M and IgG).

Treatment. Self-limited. Consider corticosteroids for visually significant subepithelial infiltrates only after infection has been ruled out.

Cytomegalovirus. Keratitis caused by the ubiquitous Cytomegalovirus (CMV) usually spread through saliva or other bodily fluids. CMV typically manifests in the cornea as an endothelitis and should be considered in cases of refractory focal or sectoral corneal edema and early graft failure.

Signs and Symptoms. Pain, photophobia, tearing, endothelitis (manifested by keratic precipitates, focal or diffuse corneal edema, endothelial cell loss), and iridocyclitis.

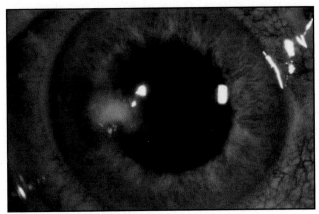

Figure 5-9. Fungal keratitis. There is a poorly demarcated corneal infiltrate with fluffy borders.

Exams and Tests. Anterior chamber paracentesis with PCR for CMV, and posterior segment examination to rule out retinitis.

Treatment. Ganciclovir (1 g PO TID) or valganciclovir (900 mg PO BID).

Fungal Keratitis

Most common in humid areas or in setting of trauma with vegetative matter or corticosteroid use. Common organisms include *Fusarium* (filamentous), *Candida* (yeast), and *Aspergillus* (filamentous) species.

Signs and Symptoms. Indolent onset of symptoms, pain, mild redness, gray-white infiltrate with feathery borders, multiple satellite lesions, endothelial plaques, anterior chamber fungal aggregate, hypopyon, and unresponsive to therapy with antibacterial agents (Figure 5-9).

Exams and Tests. Corneal scraping and culture on Sabouraud's agar or blood agar, potassium hydroxide wet mount, Giemsa stain, Gomori methenamine silver stain, calcofluor white stain.

Confocal microscopy can be used to identify filaments. Consider corneal biopsy if unresponsive to therapy with recurrent negative cultures.

Treatment. Topical natamycin 5% (starting every hour) is the drug of choice for filamentous fungi, as demonstrated by the Mycotic Ulcer Treatment Trial, while topical amphotericin B 0.15% to 0.3% is better suited to the treatment of yeast. Topical voriconazole 1% can be used as an adjunctive therapy in refractory cases. Voriconazole can also be administered via corneal intrastromal injection, intracameral injection, and intravitreal injection, depending on the depth of fungal disease. Oral fluconazole or voriconazole can be used adjunctively with local therapies. Cycloplegics can be used as needed for comfort. Steroids are contraindicated and can lead to significant escalation in disease severity.

Acanthamoeba and Other Parasitic Corneal Infections

Acanthamoeba is a parasitic infection associated with exposure to fresh water and contact lens wear with poor hygiene.

Signs and Symptoms. Severe pain (out of proportion with exam findings), photophobia, redness, indolent onset of symptoms, epithelial or subepithelial infiltrate, pseudodendrites, radial keratoneuritis (Figure 5-10), stromal ring infiltrate (Table 5-2) in late cases (beyond 3 weeks), and corneal thinning.

Exams and Tests. Corneal scrapings (Gram, Giemsa, calcofluor white, acridine orange, or periodic acid-Schiff stains), corneal culture (nonnutrient agar with *Escherichia coli* overlay), confocal microscopy to identify double-walled cysts (see Figure 2-6), and corneal biopsy.

Treatment. Topical polyhexamethylene biguanide 0.02%, chlorhexidine 0.02%, propamidine isethionate 0.1%, neomycin-polymyxin B-gramicidin every hour. Treatment will need to be continued for at least 3 months and slowly tapered. If caught early, debridement of epithelium for diagnosis can also be therapeutic.

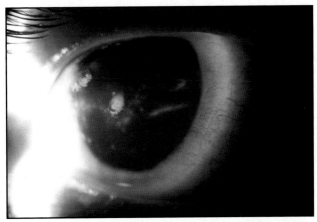

Figure 5-10. Acanthamoeba keratitis. There are multifocal epithelial infiltrates, a pseudodendritic lesion, and inflammation along the corneal nerves (radial keratoneuritis).

Table 5-2. Differential Diagnosis for Corneal Ring Infiltrates

Acanthamoeba keratitis (late finding)

Fungal keratitis

Herpes simplex virus keratitis

Pseudomonas keratitis

Topical anesthetic abuse

BIBLIOGRAPHY

1. Barron BA, Gee L, Hauck WW, et al. Herpetic Eye Disease Study. A controlled trial of oral acyclovir for herpes simplex stromal keratitis. *Ophthalmology.* 1994;101(12):1871-1882. doi:10.1016/S0161-6420(13)31155-5.

2. Weisenthal RW. *2013-2014 Basic and Clinical Science Course Section 8: External Disease and Cornea.* San Francisco, CA: American Academy of Ophthalmology; 2014.

3. Gerstenblith AT, Rabinowitz MP, eds. *The Wills Eye Manual: Office and Emergency Room Diagnosis and Treatment of Eye Disease.* Philadelphia, PA: Lippincott Williams & Wilkins; 2012.

4. Mannis MJ, Holland EJ, eds. *Cornea.* 4th ed. Edinburgh, Scotland: Elsevier Inc; 2016.

5. Prajna NV, Krishnan T, Mascarenhas J, et al. The mycotic ulcer treatment trial: a randomized trial comparing natamycin vs voriconazole. *JAMA Ophthalmol.* 2013; 131(4):422-429.

6. Srinivasan M, Mascarenhas J, Rajaraman R, et al. The Steroids for Corneal Ulcers Trial (SCUT): secondary 12-month clinical outcomes of a randomized controlled trial. *Am J Ophthalmol.* 2014;157(2):327-333.e3. doi:10.1016/j.1jo.2013.09.025.

7. Srinivasan M, Mascarenhas J, Rajaraman R, et al. Corticosteroids for bacterial keratitis: the Steroids for Corneal Ulcers Trial (SCUT). *Arch Ophthalmol.* 2012;130(2):143-150. doi:10.1001/archophthalmol.2011.315.

8. Wilhelmus KR, Dawson CR, Barron BA, et al. Risk factors for herpes simplex virus epithelial keratitis recurring during treatment of stromal keratitis or iridocyclitis. Herpetic Eye Disease Study Group. *Br J Ophthalmol.* 1996;80(11):969-972.

6

Inflammatory Conditions of the Conjunctiva and Cornea

CONJUNCTIVA

Seasonal and Perennial Allergic Conjunctivitis

Immunoglobulin (Ig)E-mediated hypersensitivity reaction that leads to release of histamines and other inflammatory mediators.

Signs and Symptoms. Bilateral itching, tearing, swelling, chemosis, injection, and papillary response with onset of symptoms immediately following exposure to allergen.

Exams and Tests. Allergic conjunctivitis is a clinical diagnosis, but consultation with allergist can be helpful to identify allergen.

Treatment. Avoidance of allergen, symptomatic relief with artificial tears and cool compresses, topical antihistamines (naphazoline, emedastine), topical mast cell stabilizers (cromolyn sodium, lodoxamide tromethamine), combination agents (olopatadine, ketotifen), topical cyclosporine 0.5%, systemic antihistamines, and topical corticosteroids in severe cases.

Kim T, Daluvoy MB.
The Pocket Guide to Cornea (pp 51-69).
© 2019 SLACK Incorporated.

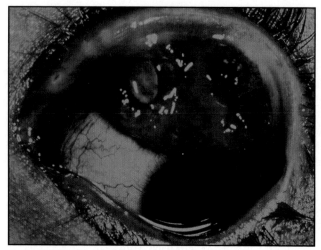

Figure 6-1. Vernal keratoconjunctivitis. Giant papillae are seen on the tarsal conjunctiva, and there is a round opacity on the cornea representing a shield ulcer.

Vernal Keratoconjunctivitis

Type I and IV hypersensitivity reactions typically affect male children seasonally.

Signs and Symptoms. Bilateral itching, thick mucoid discharge, giant papillae typically on the superior palpebral conjunctiva (Figure 6-1), conjunctival injection, chemosis, punctate epithelial erosions, pannus (usually superiorly), superior shield ulcer (noninfectious). Horner-Trantas dots are whitish collections of devitalized inflammatory cells at the limbus and are seen commonly in patients of African or Asian descent.

Exams and Tests. Clinical diagnosis.

Treatment. Topical antihistamines or topical mast cell stabilizers in mild to moderate cases; topical corticosteroids, topical cyclosporine 0.5%, or tacrolimus in severe cases. Supratarsal corticosteroid injection can also be considered.

Atopic Keratoconjunctivitis

Chronic type I hypersensitivity reaction occurs year-round and affects individuals with a history of atopy.

Signs and Symptoms. Itching, mucoid discharge, small or medium papillae on upper or lower palpebral conjunctiva, conjunctival scarring, corneal punctate epithelial erosions, eyelid crusting and eczema, predisposition to herpes simplex virus and *Staphylococcus aureus* infections.

Exams and Tests. Clinical diagnosis.

Treatment. Topical antihistamines, topical mast cell stabilizers, topical corticosteroids if severe. If disease progresses despite topical therapy, can consider systemic immunosuppression.

Giant Papillary Conjunctivitis

Hypersensitivity reaction related to soft contact lenses.

Signs and Symptoms. Itching, foreign body sensation, difficulty tolerating contact lenses, giant papillae on superior tarsal conjunctiva, high riding contact lenses, excessive movement of contact lenses, debris buildup on contact lenses.

Exams and Tests. Eversion of upper eyelid and examination for giant papillae.

Treatment. Improve contact lens fit, reduce duration of contact lens wear, more thorough cleansing of lenses including enzymatic cleaning, switch to daily disposable lenses. In severe cases, discontinue contact lenses and start topical antihistamine, mast cell stabilizer, or low-dose topical corticosteroid.

Ocular Cicatricial Pemphigoid

Also known as *mucous membrane pemphigoid*, a type II hypersensitivity reaction resulting from antibasement membrane autoantibodies.

Signs and Symptoms. Dryness, redness, conjunctival subepithelal fibrosis, forniceal foreshortening, symblepharon formation

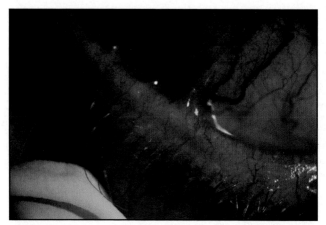

Figure 6-2. Symblepharon. Adhesions between the tarsal and bulbar conjunctiva lead to loss of the fornix.

(Figure 6-2), eyelid-globe adhesions, dry eye due to inflammatory destruction of lacrimal gland, conjunctival keratinization (Figure 6-3), entropion, trichiasis, corneal pannus, and ulceration. Oral, genital, or anal ulcerations may also occur.

Exams and Tests. Eversion of upper and lower eyelids to evaluate fibrosis and symblepharon formation, conjunctival biopsy sent in Michel solution with direct immunofluorescence or immunoperoxidase staining to demonstrate binding of complement 3, IgG, IgM, or IgA to the basement membrane. False-negative results are common.

Treatment. Doxycycline or dapsone (avoid in patients with glucose-6-phosphate dehydrogenase deficiency) for mild cases, cyclophosphamide for severe cases. Alternative immunosuppressant medications include: prednisone, rituximab, infliximab, methotrexate, azathioprine, mycophenolate mofetil, and etanercept. Epilation of eyelashes if trichiasis present, surgical correction of significant eyelid malposition, although surgery may trigger more inflammation. Eyelid margin keratinization can be treated with

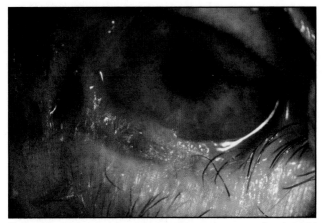

Figure 6-3. Conjunctival keratinization. Advanced stage ocular cicatricial pemphigoid with symblepharon that has become keratinized.

vitamin A ointment or excision of keratin with amniotic membrane transplantation or mucous membrane grafting. Blepharitis should be managed with warm compresses, eyelid hygiene, and doxycycline. Dry eye should be managed aggressively to prevent breakdown of the ocular surface and can be performed using a combination of preservative-free artificial tears and gel, topical cyclosporine 0.5%, lifitegrast (Xiidra, Shire), low-potency topical steroids, punctal occlusion, and serum tears. Surveillance cultures to evaluate for colonization of the ocular surface and appropriate antimicrobial therapy are also important to further limit inflammation.

Erythema Multiforme, Stevens-Johnson Syndrome, and Toxic Epidermal Necrolysis

Spectrum of type III hypersensitivity reaction to drugs or infectious diseases leading to vesiculobullous reactions on the skin and mucous membranes, with toxic epidermal necrolysis being the most severe form. The most common offending

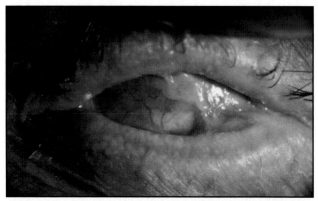

Figure 6-4. Stevens-Johnson syndrome. End stage cicatricial conjunctivitis showing symblepharon with keratinzation, obliteration of the conjunctival fornix, corneal neovascularization, and corneal opacification.

agents include sulfonamides, anticonvulsants, barbiturates, and allopurinol.

Signs and Symptoms. Rash ("target" lesion), fever, sloughing of skin, mucous membrane blisters, mucopurulent conjunctivitis, pseudo-membrane formation, episcleritis, conjunctival and corneal necrosis, ocular surface cicatrization, eyelid margin keratinization, trichiasis, entropion, and symblepharon formation (Figure 6-4).

Exams and Tests. Review systemic medications to identify cause, cultures if infection suspected, skin biopsy if diagnosis is questionable.

Treatment. Treat as thermal burn in acute phase (may require hopitalization in burn unit), discontinue offending drug, treat any underlying infections, supportive therapy with systemic hydration, preservative-free artificial tears/ointments, topical steroids or topical cyclosporine 0.5%, prophylactic topical antibiotics, amniotic membrane placement over entire ocular surface, secondary management of late sequelae such as symblepharon, eyelid malposition, and limbal stem cell disease. Systemic steroids are controversial.

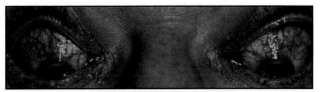

Figure 6-5. Superior limbic keratoconjunctivitis. There is localized superior hyperemia. Eversion of the upper eyelid will reveal tarsal conjunctival papillae.

Superior Limbic Keratoconjunctivitis

Recurrent bilateral inflammation resulting from mechanical trauma from the upper eyelid onto loose superior conjunctiva, usually affecting middle-aged women with thyroid dysfunction.

Signs and Symptoms. Foreign body sensation, redness, burning, hyperemia and thickening of the superior bulbar conjunctiva (Figure 6-5), redundant superior bulbar conjunctiva, fine papillae on superior tarsal conjunctiva, superior limbal hypertrophy, and filaments on the superior cornea.

Exam and Tests. Fluorescein and rose bengal staining (stains superior bulbar conjunctiva) and thyroid function tests.

Treatment. Artificial tears, punctal occlusion, topical mast cell stabilizers, large diameter bandage contact lens, cautery or resection of superior bulbar conjunctiva, silver nitrate 0.5% solution (applied via cotton tip for 10 to 20 seconds), autologous serum tears, topical cyclosporine 0.5%, acetylcysteine 10% drops if filaments are present. Many cases also self-resolve.

Ligneous Conjunctivitis

This rare disorder is caused by type I plasminogen deficiency characterized by wood-like membrane formation on the upper and lower tarsus.

Signs and Symptoms. Foreign body sensation, tearing, eyelid mass, and thick fibrinous pseudomembrane overlying conjunctiva on upper and lower tarsus (usually bilateral; Figure 6-6).

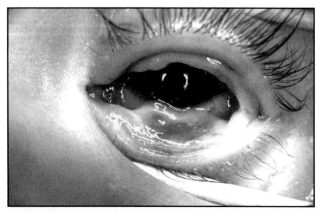

Figure 6-6. Ligneous conjunctivitis. A thick, "woody," fibrinous membrane has grown along the tarsus and eyelid margins.

Exams and Tests. Genetic testing for mutations in the plasminogen gene is recommended.

Treatment. Surgical removal of fibrinous membrane (though typically recur), adjunctive cryotherapy, topical cyclosporine 0.5%, topical corticosteroids, systemic administration of plasminogen , topical fresh frozen plasma, topical heparin, or topical plasminogen (unavailable in the United States). Can also self-resolve after months or years.

CORNEA

Interstitial Keratitis

Type IV hypersensitivity reaction resulting in corneal stromal infiltration. Common etiologies include herpes simplex virus, varicella zoster virus, congenital or acquired syphilis, tuberculosis, leprosy, Lyme disease, Epstein-Barr virus, and Cogan syndrome (vertigo, hearing loss, and stromal keratitis).

Signs and Symptoms. Pain, tearing, sectoral redness, bilateral involvement, stromal infiltrate (nonsuppurative), corneal neovascularization, iridocyclitis, keratic precipitates, and corneal edema. Signs of previous episode include deep stromal haze/scarring and ghost vessels.

Exams and Tests. Workup for underlying etiology (listed previously) depends on systemic symptoms and signs.

Treatment. Treatment of underlying etiology, topical corticosteroids (prednisolone 1% or dexamethasone 0.1%) every 2 to 4 hours; if cycloplegic, consider referral to internist or infectious disease specialist to evaluate underlying cause.

Thygeson Superficial Punctate Keratitis

Chronic recurrent punctate keratopathy possibly of viral or immunopathologic etiology.

Signs and Symptoms. Foreign body sensation, photophobia, tearing, multiple elevated clusters of gray-white epithelial lesions that demonstrate negative staining, and lack of conjunctival findings (Figure 6-7).

Exams and Tests. Slit-lamp examination with fluorescein staining.

Treatment. Artificial tears are recommended in most cases; if persitent or severe, can use low-potency topical steroid, topical cyclosporine 0.5% or 2%, topical tacrolimus solution 0.02%, or bandage contact lenses for comfort.

Neurotrophic Keratitis

Corneal hypoesthesia with multiple causes (Table 6-1), most commonly herpetic keratitis, topical medication toxicity, diabetic neuropathy, or damage to the trigeminal nerve. Sequelae include persistent corneal epithelial defects, corneal neovascularization, and opacification.

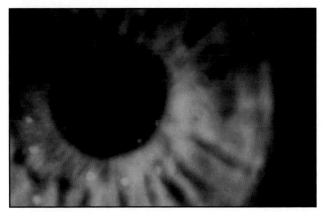

Figure 6-7. Thygeson superficial punctate keratitis. There are multiple gray-white epithelial opacities.

Signs and Symptoms. Foreign body sensation, redness, reduced corneal sensation, persistent corneal epithelial defect commonly with rolled edges, and corneal ulcer (Figure 6-8).

Exams and Tests. Corneal sensation testing prior to application of topical anesthetic, and slit-lamp examination with fluorescein staining; consider neuroimaging if there is concern for central nervous system lesion.

Treatment. Aggressive lubrication with preservative-free artificial tears/ointment, punctal occlusion, autologous serum drops, bandage contact lens, and discontinuation of preservative-containing topical medications. If severe, consider amniotic membrane, tarsorrhaphy, or conjunctival flap.

Phlyctenular Keratoconjunctivitis

Type IV hypersensitivity reaction to microbial antigens (most commonly *Staphylococcus* and tuberculosis) resulting in corneal and conjunctival inflammation.

Table 6-1. Differential Diagnosis for Persistent Corneal Epithelial Defect

Abnormal eyelid position or function

    Floppy eyelid syndrome

    Lower eyelid ectropion or entropion

    Lagophthalmos

    Trichiasis

Keratoconjunctivitis sicca

Limbal stem cell deficiency

Neurotrophic keratitis

    Diabetes

    Herpetic

    Nerve damage

Ocular surface irregularities

    Band keratopathy

    Dellen

    Salzmann nodule

Toxicity from topical medications

Trauma

Signs and Symptoms. Foreign body sensation, redness, tearing, or small elevated nodules adjacent to engorged vessels (Figure 6-9) may be present, usually at the limbus, conjunctiva, or cornea.

Exams and Tests. Evaluate for *Staphylococcal blepharitis*, rule out tuberculosis; culture if suspicious for infection.

Treatment. Treat underlying blepharitis or infection, antibiotic ointment, topical corticosteroids QID, oral doxycycline or tetracycline.

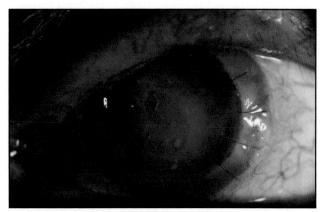

Figure 6-8. Non-healing epithelial defect. A persistent neurotrophic ulcer with rolled borders is stained with fluorescein.

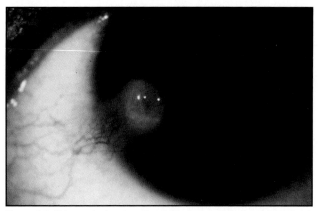

Figure 6-9. Phlyctenular keratoconjunctivitis. A vascularized nodular lesion is seen on the cornea.

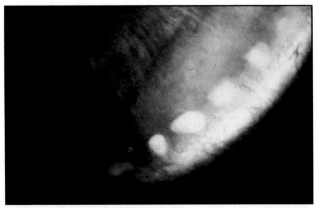

Figure 6-10. Staphylococcal marginal keratitis. There are multiple limbal infiltrates with intervening clear zones in a hypersensitivity reaction to *Staphylococcus*.

Staphylococcal Marginal Keratitis

Corneal infiltrates near the limbus as a hypersensitivity reaction to *Staphylococcus* (inflammation, not infection).

Signs and Symptoms. Pain, foreign body sensation, photophobia, small round infiltrates 1 mm inside the limbus often located at the 2, 4, 8, or 10 o'clock positions (where eyelid margin contacts the limbus), intervening clear zone between limbus and infiltrate, history of recurrent episodes (Figure 6-10).

Exams and Tests. Slit-lamp examination with fluorescein staining (infiltrates demonstrate variable staining) should be performed; culture if suspicion for infection or first episode.

Treatment. Eyelid hygiene (warm compresses, eyelid scrubs), antibiotic drop or ointment BID-QID; after infection has been ruled out, start either low-dose topical corticosteroid or steroid/antibiotic combination. If recurrent, add oral doxycycline or tetracycline.

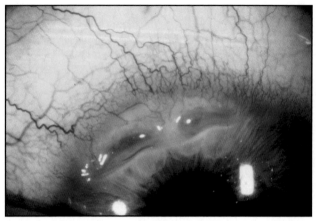

Figure 6-11. Mooren's ulcer. Corneal melting is observed at the peripheral cornea with associated conjunctival hyperemia.

Mooren's Ulcer

Inflammatory ulceration of the peripheral cornea, not associated with systemic collagen vascular diseases. A more aggressive form exists in Africa with rapid progression, lack of response to treatment, and possible association with parasitic infections.

Signs and Symptoms. Severe pain, redness, photophobia, peripheral corneal infiltrate or melt that spreads circumferentially then centrally with a leading edge of devitalized tissue (Figure 6-11), lack of scleral involvement.

Exams and Tests. Slit-lamp examination to determine degree of stromal thinning, fluorescein staining (epithelial defect usually present), rheumatologic consultation to rule out underlying systemic autoimmune disease (distinguishes from peripheral ulcerative keratitis). This is a diagnosis of exclusion.

Treatment. Antibiotic ointment, bandage contact lens, amniotic membrane, topical collagenase inhibitors (medroxyprogesterone 1%, acetylcysteine 10%), topical cyclosporine 2%, topical interferon alpha, tarsorrhaphy, local conjunctival resection

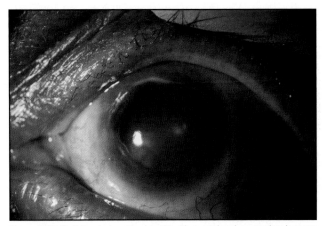

Figure 6-12. Peripheral ulcerative keratitis. The peripheral cornea has become ulcerated in association with an underlying systemic autoimmune disease.

to reduce inflow of inflammatory mediators. Cautious use of topical corticosteroids. Systemic immunosuppression may be beneficial (common agents include cyclophosphamide, methotrexate, and topical cyclosporine 0.5%).

Peripheral Ulcerative Keratitis

Ulceration of the peripheral cornea in patients with a history of systemic autoimmune disease, such as rheumatoid arthritis, systemic lupus erythematosus, polyarteritis nodosa, Wegener granulomatosis, and ulcerative colitis.

Signs and Symptoms. Pain, foreign body sensation, redness, peripheral corneal infiltrate or melt (usually limited to one sector); can have scleral involvement (Figure 6-12).

Exams and Tests. Slit-lamp examination to determine degree of stromal thinning, fluorescein staining (epithelial defect usually present), and rheumatologic consultation for evaluation and treatment of underlying systemic autoimmune disease.

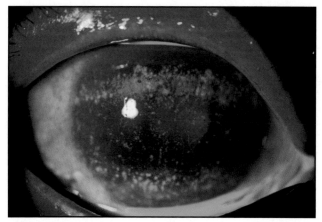

Figure 6-13. Keratoconjunctivitis sicca. Nearly confluent epithelial erosions are highlighted with fluorescein staining.

Treatment. Systemic immunosuppression is the mainstay of treatment (common agents include cyclophosphamide, methotrexate, and topical cyclosporine 0.5%) with systemic corticosteroid bridge. Adjunctive local therapies include preservative-free artificial tears, antibiotic ointment, bandage contact lenses, amniotic membrane, collagenase inhibitors (medroxyprogesterone 1%, acetylcysteine 10%), topical cyclosporine 2%, tarsorrhaphy, and local conjunctival resection to reduce inflow of inflammatory mediators. Topical corticosteroids must be used with caution to avoid infection and stromal melt.

Ocular Graft Versus Host Disease

Complication after allogeneic hematopoietic stem cell transplantation wherein the grafted cells attack the host cells.

Signs and Symptoms. Foreign body sensation, irritation, redness, keratoconjunctivitis sicca (Figure 6-13), conjunctival chemosis, conjunctival scarring, cicatrization, limbal stem cell deficiency, and secondary corneal scarring.

Exams and Tests. Slit-lamp examination with lissamine green or fluorescein staining, Schirmer's testing, or tear composition assays.

Treatment. Aggressive lubrication with preservative-free artificial tears/ointment, punctal occlusion, topical cyclosporine 0.5%, autologous serum tears, amniotic membrane, and scleral contact lenses. Systemic therapy may need to be increased if ocular disease cannot be controlled with topical medication alone.

OTHER INFLAMMATORY DISORDERS INVOLVING THE OCULAR SURFACE

Episcleritis

Inflammation of the episclera is usually idiopathic but can be associated with systemic inflammatory conditions (collagen vascular disease, rosacea, gout, thyroid dysfunction). Episcleritis can be simple (localized or diffuse) or nodular (associated with formation of slightly tender, mobile nodule).

Signs and Symptoms. Redness, mild soreness, or superficial episcleral hyperemia might be present.

Exams and Tests. Application of 2.5% phenylephrine (will produce blanching of episcleral vessels but not scleral vessels after 15 minutes); movement of episclera with cotton-tip applicator confirms level of inflammation. Consider workup for underlying inflammatory condition if multiple recurrences.

Treatment. Generally self-limited. Artificial tears, topical or systemic nonsteroidal anti-inflammatory drugs (NSAIDs) for symptomatic relief, short course of low-potency topical corticosteroids if severe or unresponsive.

Scleritis

Immune-mediated scleral inflammation is associated with an underlying systemic inflammatory condition, most commonly rheumatoid arthritis.

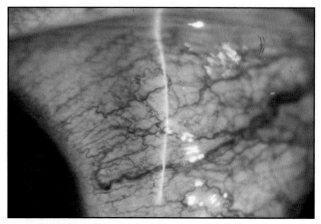

Figure 6-14. Scleritis. There is scleral hyperemia with an elevated nodule that does not blanch with phenylephrine.

Nonnecrotizing: Diffuse or Nodular

Signs and Symptoms. Deep boring pain, violaceous scleral hyperemia that does not blanch with phenylephrine, tender immobile solitary scleral nodule, avascular and edematous patch of sclera (Figure 6-14).

Exams and Tests. Systemic workup for autoimmune diseases, infections (tuberculosis, leprosy, syphilis, Lyme disease, Bartonella, and herpes zoster), and gout.

Treatment. Systemic NSAIDs (ibuprofen 800 mg PO TID or naproxen 500 mg PO BID, indomethacin 25 mg PO TID), topical high-potency corticosteroids, or subconjunctival corticosteroids. Consider systemic corticosteroids or immunosuppressive therapy if unresponsive.

Necrotizing. With or without inflammation (scleromalacia perforans).

Signs and Symptoms. Deep pain but can be asymptomatic in scleromalacia perforans, bluish hue to the sclera, scleral thinning, exposure of uveal tissue, and globe rupture with minimal trauma.

Exam and Tests. Same as for nonnecrotizing scleritis.

Treatment. Systemic immunosuppression with corticosteroid bridge, scleral patch graft if impending perforation. Periocular corticosteroids should be avoided as these can exacerbate scleral thinning.

BIBLIOGRAPHY

1.　Shikari H, Antin JH, Dana R. Ocular graft-versus-host disease: a review. *Surv Ophthalmol.* 2013;58(3):233-251.

2.　O'Brien T. Allergic conjunctivitis: an update on diagnosis and management. *Curr Opin Allergy Clin Immunol.* 2013;13(5):543-549. doi:10.1097/ACI.0b013e328364ec3a.

3.　Queisi MM, Zein M, Lamba N, Meese H, Foster CS. Update on ocular cicatricial pemphigoid and emerging treatments. *Surv Ophthalmol.* 2016;61(3):314-317. doi:10.1016/j.survophthal.2015.12.007.

4.　Mannis MJ, Holland EJ, eds. *Cornea.* 4th ed. Edinburgh, Scotland: Elsevier Inc; 2016.

5.　Weisenthal RW. *2013-2014 Basic and Clinical Science Course Section 8: External Disease and Cornea.* San Francisco, CA: American Academy of Ophthalmology; 2014.

6.　Gerstenblith AT, Rabinowitz MP, eds. *The Wills Eye Manual: Office and Emergency Room Diagnosis and Treatment of Eye Disease.* Philadelphia, PA: Lippincott Williams & Wilkins; 2012.

7

Neoplasms

Epithelial Tumors

Conjunctival Squamous Papilloma

Fleshy lesions of the conjunctiva characterized by a central vascular core surrounded by numerous capillaries and covered by a translucent squamous epithelium. Can be sessile (flat) or pedunculated (Figure 7-1).

Signs and Symptoms. Asymptomatic or may cause surface irritation. Squamous papillomas rarely undergo malignant transformation, but involvement of the palpebral conjunctiva, inflammation, and symblepharon may indicate dysplasia. Lesions appearing in clusters may be indicative of human papillomavirus (HPV) infection, typically of subtype 6, 11, 16, 18, or 33.

Exams and Tests. Slit-lamp examination, excision allows for histopathologic examination, often demonstrating acanthotic, nonkeratinizing squamous epithelium. Polymerase chain reaction can indicate whether an HPV subtype is associated with a lesion.

Kim T, Daluvoy MB.
The Pocket Guide to Cornea (pp 71-91).
© 2019 SLACK Incorporated.

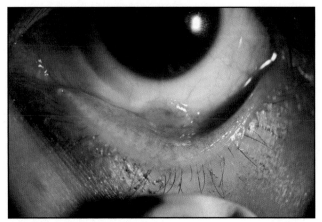

Figure 7-1. Conjunctival squamous papilloma. A fleshy lesion is seen in the lower forniceal conjunctiva with a central vascular core surrounded by capillaries and covered with a translucent epithelium.

Treatment. Simple excision with cryotherapy to the lesion base and adjacent conjunctiva may be performed, but recurrence and seeding is common. Adjuvant medical therapies used with success include intralesional and topical interferon alpha-2b, topical mitomycin C, and oral cimetidine.

Hereditary Benign Intraepithelial Dyskeratosis

Also known as HBID, this autosomal dominant disorder affects the Haliwa-Saponi Native American tribe, historically located in the Halifax and Washington counties of North Carolina, USA. HBID is associated with a gene duplication at location 4q35.

Signs and Symptoms. Patients often begin to manifest conjunctival lesions within the first decade of life. The lesions are characterized by a keratinized, elevated appearance extending along the limbus and surrounding conjunctival injection (Figure 7-2). Patients report redness, photophobia, and foreign body sensation.

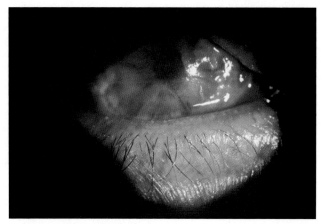

Figure 7-2. HBID. Keratinized plaques covering the corneal and conjunctival surface are seen.

Extension of plaques onto the corneal surface leads to decreased vision.

Exams and Tests. Slit-lamp examination of a patient with appropriate history is typically sufficient to identify these lesions. Histopathologic examination demonstrates acanthosis, parakeratosis, and dyskeratosis with a chronic inflammatory cell infiltrate.

Treatment. Lesions may be treated with simple excision, but recurrence is common. Lubrication and topical steroids may also be used for symptom control but will not cause regression of lesions.

Ocular Surface Squamous Neoplasia

Ocular surface squamous neoplasia (OSSN) is dysplastic squamous epithelium of the cornea and/or conjunctiva. OSSN is an umbrella term encompassing the terms conjunctival/corneal intraepithelial neoplasia and invasive squamous cell carcinoma (SCC).

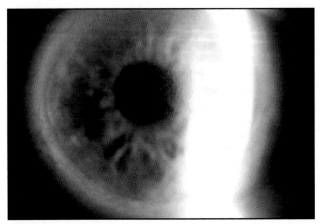

Figure 7-3. Corneal intraepithelial neoplasia. The patient demonstrates a sectoral frosting of the epithelium.

Conjunctival Intraepithelial Neoplasia.

Conjunctival intraepithelial neoplasia (CIN) is a dysplastic lesion of the squamous epithelium of the conjunctiva that does not invade the epithelial basement membrane.

Signs and Symptoms. Typically, asymptomatic and found incidentally on examination or because of patient concern for cosmetic appearance. As opposed to the vascular "dot pattern" of benign squamous papilloma, the vascular pattern of CIN involves fine branching vessels with a "hairpin" configuration. Lesions themselves typically have a gelatinous appearance and are slowly progressive. Corneal involvement is indicated by areas of frosted epithelium and/or pannus (Figure 7-3).

Exams and Tests. Slit-lamp examination aids. A stippled staining pattern with fluorescein or rose bengal supports the possibility of dysplasia. Confirmation of the diagnosis requires biopsy. Histopathology demonstrates dysplasia of the conjunctival epithelium (indicated by high nuclear to cytoplasmic ratio, disorganization, and mitotic figures at any epithelial level) with an intact basement membrane. High-resolution anterior segment optical coherence tomography (OCT) demonstrates a thickened, hyperreflective epithelium, with an abrupt transition between normal and abnormal epithelium. Confocal microscopy can also be used to help in diagnosis.

Treatment. Depending on size and location, lesions can be treated medically, surgically, or with a combination of both medical and surgical therapy. Topical chemotherapy agents include 5-fluorouracil, interferon alpha-2b, and mitomycin C. Interferon alpha-2b can also be injected intralesionally, particularly for superior forniceal lesions that may not be amenable to topical therapy. New lesions can also be excised using the "no-touch" technique, removing at least 2 mm margins down to bare sclera with cryotherapy applied to the conjunctival borders. Involved cornea is simultaneously debrided, often with alcohol epitheliectomy. Recurrence of lesions can occur in 30% to 50% of cases and tend to be more invasive, thus warranting more aggressive treatment. Recurrent lesions are typically treated with wide excision with or without mitomycin C and aggressive cryotherapy. Extensive limbal resection may increase the risk of development of limbal stem cell deficiency and may warrant later treatment with limbal autograft.

Invasive Squamous Cell Carcinoma. Invasive squamous SCC refers to the penetration of dysplastic epithelium beyond the epithelial basement membrane. CIN is thought to be a precursor to SCC lesions.

Signs and Symptoms. SCC lesions are typically classified by appearance as gelatinous, leukoplakic, or papilliform, but significant overlap exists between these subtypes. Invasion of SCC is indicated by adherence to the underlying episclera and sclera and the presence of feeder vessels. Affected areas of cornea are often indicated by a frosted appearance or the presence of fibrovascular pannus (Figure 7-4).

Exams and Tests. Slit-lamp examination to identify concerning lesions. Deep tissue adherence and the presence of feeder vessels may be indicative of malignancy. Affected areas of corneal

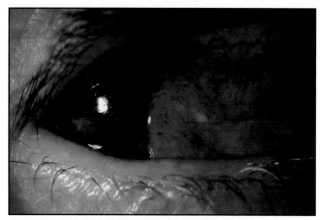

Figure 7-4. Invasive squamous cell carcinoma. A large gelatinous lesion with several feeder vessels involving both the cornea and conjunctiva is seen.

epithelium can be identified with fluorescein and rose bengal staining. Histopathologic evaluation demonstrates penetration of dysplastic cells through the epithelial basement membrane. Invasion is typically limited to the conjunctival portion of lesions, as Bowman's layer appears to prevent penetration into the corneal stroma. High-resolution anterior segment OCT can be used for diagnosis, as discussed for CIN above. Confocal microscopy can demonstrate changes in cellular morphology of SCC lesions. Depth of ocular invasion may be assessed using ultrasound biomicroscopy (UBM).

Treatment. Wide local excision in a "no-touch technique" with 2 mm to 4 mm margins and double freeze-thaw cryotherapy to the excision margins and limbus is indicated for SCC. A lamellar sclerectomy may be needed if scleral involvement is apparent. Corneal epitheliectomy is also performed to address involved areas of cornea, while taking special care to avoid penetration of Bowman's layer because of its barrier properties. Chemotherapeutic agents are often used as adjuvants, including topical interferon alpha-2b, mitomycin C, and 5-fluorouracil. Use of adjuvant chemotherapy reduces recurrence rates after resection from approximately 40% to 10%. Extensive local invasion may require enucleation or exenteration. Regional and systemic metastasis is rare, with mortality ranging between 0% and 8%.

Mucoepidermoid Carcinoma

A highly aggressive form of SCC, mucoepidermoid carcinoma (MEC) has a propensity for invasion of the globe and orbit.

Signs and Symptoms. Appearance is similar to that of typical SCC, but MEC may arise from the caruncle. It is typically locally invasive at the time of diagnosis.

Exams and Tests. Slit-lamp examination to identify concerning lesions. Affected areas of corneal epithelium can be identified with fluorescein and rose bengal staining. Histopathologic evaluation demonstrates penetration of dysplastic cells through the epithelial basement membrane as well as mucin-producing goblet cells. Confocal microscopy can demonstrate changes in cellular morphology of MEC lesions. Depth of ocular invasion may be assessed using UBM.

Treatment. MEC is typically managed with wide local excision and aggressive cryotherapy. Intraocular spread may require enucleation because of high rate of regional lymph node metastasis. Orbital spread typically requires exenteration with or without sentinel lymph node biopsy.

GLANDULAR TUMORS

Sebaceous Cell Carcinoma

Typically originates in the Meibomian or Zeis glands, spreading in an intraepithelial (pagetoid) manner to involve the ocular surface. There is some evidence that sebaceous cell carcinoma may also originate within the tarsal conjunctiva (Figure 7-5).

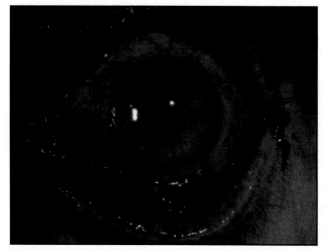

Figure 7-5. Sebaceous cell carcinoma. This external photo demonstrates a sebaceous cell lesion involving the inferior tarsal conjunctiva.

Signs and Symptoms. Conjunctival sebaceous cell carcinoma often presents as a unilateral blepharoconjunctivitis. It is characterized by unilateral injection and pannus and may be associated with eyelid margin thickening and eyelash loss (madarosis).

Exams and Tests. Slit-lamp appearance can be misleading, as sebaceous cell carcinoma of the conjunctiva may masquerade as several other conditions, including blepharitis, chalazion, or superior limbic keratoconjunctivitis. Unilateral findings associated with eyelid involvement that does not resolve with appropriate treatment should prompt consideration of sebaceous cell carcinoma. Biopsy is necessary to confirm the diagnosis. Histopathologic examination demonstrates anaplastic superficial epithelial cells with normal deeper epithelial layers (in contrast to SCC, in which dysplasia is typically found both in deep and superficial layers).

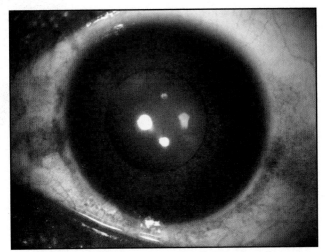

Figure 7-6. Benign acquired melanosis. This slit-lamp photo demonstrates benign conjunctival pigmentation that has increased with age.

Treatment. If the diagnosis of sebaceous cell carcinoma is confirmed, map biopsy is warranted to determine the extent of disease involvement. If more than 50% of the ocular surface is involved, exenteration is indicated. Less extensive disease may be treated with wide local excision and aggressive cryotherapy to excision margins. Sentinel lymph node biopsy may be helpful in staging.

NEUROECTODERMAL TUMORS

Benign Acquired Melanosis

A unilateral or bilateral increase in conjunctival pigmentation, typically secondary to genetic, toxic, or metabolic factors. As the name indicates, such melanosis does not confer an increased risk of melanoma.

Signs and Symptoms. Bilateral increases in pigmentation are typically seen in darkly pigmented individuals with age (Figure 7-6). They may also be seen in patients with metabolic disorders or toxic exposures.

Exams and Tests. Serial slit-lamp examinations are warranted to confirm the diagnosis. Concern for pigmented lesions with neoplastic potential may warrant biopsy to confirm the diagnosis. Slit-lamp photos may establish a baseline for future comparison of exam findings.

Treatment. No treatment is necessary for this benign condition.

Ocular Melanocytosis

Also referred to as *subepithelial congenital melanosis*, a condition involving a congenital increase in quantity of pigmented melanocytes in the sclera and episclera, as well as within the uvea.

Signs and Symptoms. Presentation is typically at birth, characterized by a unilateral scleral/episcleral pigmentation and ipsilateral heavily pigmented iris (resulting in iris heterochromia). Association of ocular melanocytosis with ipsilateral dermal melanosis of the facial skin is referred to as *oculodermal melanocytosis* (or *nevus of Ota*). Oculodermal melanocytosis is most frequently seen in patients of Asian or African descent.

Exams and Tests. External and slit-lamp examination is typically sufficient.

Treatment. No treatment is required. There is a slightly increased risk of uveal melanoma in patients with ocular melanocytosis, but no prophylactic therapeutic intervention exists.

Ephelis

Ephelis (or freckle) is a pigmented lesion of the conjunctival epithelium without malignant potential.

Signs and Symptoms. An ephelis is typically seen at birth or in childhood. It is characterized by a pigmented appearance of a region of conjunctiva secondary to an excess of melanin production within the basal epithelium despite having a normal density of melanocytes. During puberty, these lesions may increase in pigmentation slightly, and may be more readily noticed.

Exams and Tests. Slit-lamp examination is typically sufficient. Slit-lamp photos may establish a baseline for future comparison.

Treatment. No treatment is necessary for this benign lesion. It may occasionally be excised for cosmesis.

Nevus

A benign noncancerous collection of nevus cells that is classified by its location (junctional, subepithelial, or compound).

Signs and Symptoms. Nevi appear as pigmented lesions that may be flat (junctional) or elevated (subepithelial or compound). Pigmentation may increase or growth of lesions may occur during puberty or pregnancy, making them more readily noticeable (Figure 7-7A). They can also lack pigment (Figure 7-7B).

Exams and Tests. Slit-lamp examination. Histopathologic examination may demonstrate epithelial inclusions within nevi, with associated cystic spaces. Pigmentation varies from amelanotic to heavily pigmented.

Treatment. These lesions are typically observed long-term, with photos obtained to establish a baseline appearance. As melanoma can arise from a preexisting nevus, development of features concerning for malignancy (increased thickness, feeder vessels, variation in pigmentation, irregular borders) should be monitored with complete excision and histopathologic evaluation if they develop.

Primary Acquired Melanosis

Primary acquired melanosis (PAM) is a pigmented melanocytic lesion of the conjunctiva with the potential for malignant transformation.

Signs and Symptoms. PAM typically presents in the fifth or sixth decade of life as a stippled flat pigmentation of the conjunctival epithelium (typically the temporal or inferior bulbar conjunctiva). PAM can occur with or without atypia and is only distinguished histopathologically (Figure 7-8). Only PAM with atypia has malignant potential. Risk factors for malignant transformation

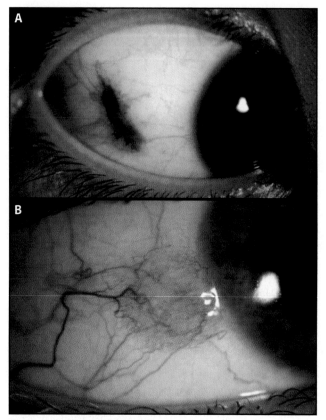

Figure 7-7. Nevi. (A) Demonstrates an elevated pigmented nevus. (B) Demonstrates a flat amelanotic nevus.

include increased thickness and greater extent in clock hours. Up to one-third of PAM lesions progress to melanoma, demonstrating the need for careful histologic evaluation for risk stratification.

Exams and Tests. Slit-lamp examination can identify the presence of a PAM lesion but may not reveal its full extent. Use of ultraviolet light or confocal microscopy may better identify the extent of

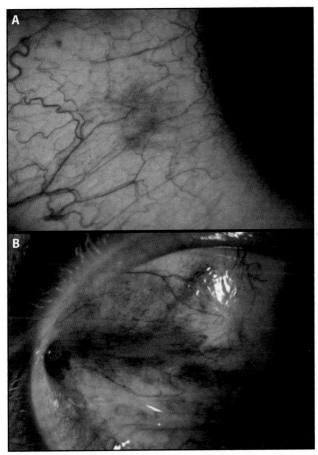

Figure 7-8. PAM. (A) Demonstrates a PAM lesion without atypia on biopsy. (B) Demonstrates a PAM lesion with atypia on biopsy.

involved conjunctival tissue. Histopathologic evaluation can demonstrate varied features from lesion to lesion. Melanocytes may have varying degrees of atypia and morphologies. The extent of epithelial involvement and invasion pattern can be useful prognostic factors. In particular, pagetoid spread (a lateral spread within the epithelium without elevation of surface tissue) confers a 90% risk of progression to melanoma.

Treatment. Lesions concerning for PAM require biopsy to confirm the diagnosis. Biopsy can be performed using an incisional, excisional, or map technique. Cryotherapy may or may not be applied to margins depending on clinical suspicion. For lesions with moderate to severe atypia, topical mitomycin C or interferon alpha-2b may be considered.

Conjunctival Melanoma

A malignant melanocytic lesion of the ocular surface that may arise from PAM, nevi, or de novo.

Signs and Symptoms. Conjunctival melanoma typically presents in Caucasian adults. It is exceedingly rare in children and in darkly pigmented individuals. In two-thirds of cases, melanoma arises from PAM, indicating the importance of biopsy and histopathologic examination of PAM lesions. Lesions of the conjunctiva demonstrating increasing thickness and increasing extent in clock hours raise concern for melanoma (Figure 7-9). While commonly pigmented, melanoma of the ocular surface can also be amelanotic, and requires high clinical suspicion for timely diagnosis.

Exams and Tests. Slit-lamp examination can demonstrate a nodular, diffusely pigmented, or amelanotic lesion. It is often associated with PAM or nevi. Histopathologic examination demonstrates melanocytes exhibiting atypia (large cells with prominent nucleoli and high nuclear-to-cytoplasmic ratio, with frequent mitotic figures) invading subepithelial tissues. Amelanotic lesions may require immunohistochemical staining such as human melanoma black 45, MELAN-A, or S-100 for confirmation of a melanocytic origin.

Treatment. Lesions suspicious for conjunctival melanoma require wide excision (at least 4 mm margins) using a dry "no-touch" technique and cryotherapy to the conjunctival margins.

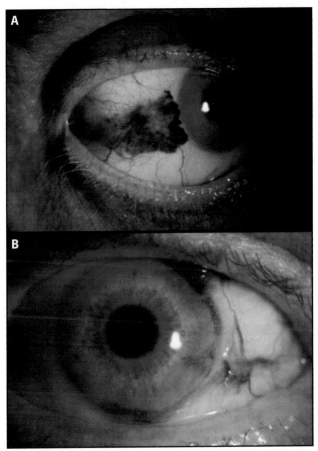

Figure 7-9. Conjunctival melanoma. (A) Demonstrates a conjunctival melanoma with diffuse pigmentation. (B) Demonstrates a multifocal nodular conjunctival melanoma.

"No-touch" refers to the manipulation of only conjunctiva thought to be normal and not the lesion itself given the theoretic risk of tumor seeding. The affected cornea should be treated with alcohol epitheliectomy without damaging Bowman's layer. Sclera suspected of involvement may be removed with lamellar sclerectomy. Recurrences should be treated surgically as well. Sentinel lymph node biopsy may help with staging for micrometastasis in patients without distant disease, but the utility of this procedure is not certain. Intraocular or intraorbital extension may occur, and may require enucleation or exenteration, respectively.

VASCULAR AND MESENCHYMAL TUMORS

Capillary Hemangioma

A lobular vascular lesion of the conjunctiva.

Signs and Symptoms. Conjunctival capillary hemangiomas may present at any age, and appear as reddish, elevated lesions that may protrude from the ocular surface.

Exams and Tests. Slit-lamp examination is typically sufficient to identify this lesion. It is distinguished from pyogenic granuloma by an intact surface epithelium over the lesion and a regular lobular architecture.

Treatment. If symptomatic, conjunctival capillary hemangiomas may be managed with excision or cryotherapy.

Pyogenic Granuloma

A proliferation of granulation tissue and vascular endothelial cells. Contrary to what the name pyogenic granuloma indicates, it does not involve granulomatous inflammation or infection.

Signs and Symptoms. Often presents in response to a traumatic, surgical, or inflammatory insult. The lesions grow rapidly, are pedunculated, and bleed easily.

Exams and Tests. Slit-lamp examination may be sufficient. Confirmation of diagnosis can be obtained with excisional biopsy. Histopathologic evaluation demonstrates immature capillaries, a myxoid interstitium, and absence of surface epithelium.

Treatment. Pyogenic granuloma can be treated with topical or intralesional steroid injection or excision and cautery of the base. Primary closure of the surrounding conjunctiva is helpful in preventing recurrence.

Kaposi Sarcoma

The most common tumor occurring in patients with HIV, Kaposi sarcoma is caused by human herpesvirus 8. It affects the conjunctiva in 20% of patients.

Signs and Symptoms. Lesions are often nodular or diffuse, and typically involve the inferior fornix.

Exams and Tests. Slit-lamp examination and historical context are typically sufficient to identify this lesion. Biopsy may aid in diagnosis in equivocal cases.

Treatment. Observation. Improvement of immune status with antiretroviral therapy may aid in disease control. Local radiation and cryotherapy may also aid in disease control.

LYMPHATIC AND LYMPHOCYTIC TUMORS

Lymphangioma

A collection of lymphatic channel elements analogous to a capillary hemangioma.

Signs and Symptoms. Typically present at birth and may demonstrate slow growth. Patients may present with the finding of an edematous patch of cysts on the conjunctiva or may present because of growth of the lesion with a systemic condition such as an upper respiratory infection. Intralesional hemorrhage

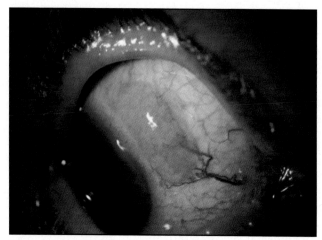

Figure 7-10. Conjunctival lymphoma. This slit-lamp photo demonstrates a salmon-colored, fleshy, vascularized lymphoma of the conjunctiva.

may result in the appearance of rapid growth and gives a classic "chocolate cyst" appearance to the lesion.

Exams and Tests. Slit-lamp examination may be sufficient. In some cases, differentiation from conjunctival capillary hemangioma requires excisional biopsy.

Treatment. Symptomatic lesions are typically managed with simple excision. Likelihood of recurrence is generally low.

Lymphoid Hyperplasia and Lymphoma

Essentially indistinguishable on clinical examination and arise from collections of lymphocytes within conjunctival tissue. Patients with either condition may develop systemic lymphoma.

Signs and Symptoms. Typically present after the age of 40 years (or in the setting of immunosuppression at a younger age) with a salmon-colored, fleshy, mobile, vascularized lesion of the conjunctiva (Figure 7-10). At the time of diagnosis, systemic lymphoma is typically not present.

Exams and Tests. Slit-lamp examination is typically sufficient but cannot distinguish between lymphoid hyperplasia and lymphoma. Histopathologic examination is essential, as morphologic features of involved cells are helpful in determining prognosis. Lymphoid tumors are typically divided into small-cell, intermediate-cell, and large-cell lesions. Small-cell lesions are well differentiated, with mature monotonous lymphocytes. Large-cell lesions contain anaplastic cells with cleaved nuclei. Large-cell lesions are more likely to be associated with extraocular disease than small-cell and intermediate-cell lesions. Immunohistochemistry may also be performed, which can differentiate between polyclonal lymphoid hyperplasia (approximately one-quarter of lesions), monoclonal B-cell lymphoma (nearly three-quarters of lesions), and other, rarer forms of lymphoid lesions. T-cell lymphomas and Hodgkin lymphomas are rarely seen in the conjunctiva. The distinction between polyclonal lymphoid hyperplasia and monoclonal B-cell lymphoma has not been demonstrated to be helpful in determining prognosis in individual patients. Extensive disease and location in the forniceal or midbulbar conjunctiva are risk factors for development of systemic lymphoma.

Treatment. Patients with biopsy-confirmed lymphoid lesions require evaluation for systemic disease, including lymph node palpation, whole-body computed tomography, bone marrow biopsy, extensive serologic testing, bone scan, and liver-spleen scan. Disease confined to the conjunctiva is treated with radiation. Cryotherapy may be of use in small, accessible lesions. Intralesional interferon alpha-2b may also be considered. Patients with systemic disease require management by a medical oncologist. Regular follow-up is required for all patients with biopsy-confirmed lymphoid lesions, as systemic disease can develop many years after presentation.

BIBLIOGRAPHY

1. Hawkins AS, Yu J, Hamming NA, Rubenstein JB. Treatment of recurrent conjunctival papillomatosis with mitomycin C. *Am J Ophthalmol.* 1999;128(5):638-640.

2. Schechter BA, Rand WJ, Velazquez GE, Williams WD, Starasoler L. Treatment of conjunctival papillomata with topical interferon Alfa-2b. *Am J Ophthalmol.* 2002;134(2):268-270. doi:10.1016/S000-9394(02)01514-3.

3. Reed JW, Cashwell F, Klintworth GK. Corneal manifestations of hereditary benign intraepithelial dyskeratosis. *Arch Ophthalmol.* 1979;97(2):297-300.

4. Yanoff M. Hereditary benign intraepithelial dyskeratosis. *Arch Ophthalmol.* 1968;79(3):291-293.

5. Erie JC, Campbell RJ, Liesegang TJ. Conjunctival and corneal intraepithelial and invasive neoplasia. *Ophthalmology.* 1986;93(2):176-183. doi:10.1016/S0161-6420(86)33764-3.

6. Waring GO 3rd, Roth AM, Ekins MB. Clinical and pathologic description of 17 cases of corneal intraepithelial neoplasia. *Am J Ophthalmol.* 1984;97(5):547-559.

7. Frucht-Pery J, Rozenman Y. Mitomycin C therapy for corneal intraepithelial neoplasia. *Am J Ophthalmol.* 1994;117(2):164-168.

8. Odrich MG, Jakobiec FA, Lancaster WD, et al. A spectrum of bilateral squamous conjunctival tumors associated with human papillomavirus type 16. *Ophthalmology.* 1991;98(5):628-635. doi:10.1016/S0161-6420(91)32218-8.

9. Fraunfelder FT, Wingfield D. Management of intraepithelial conjunctival tumors and squamous cell carcinomas. *Am J Ophthalmol.* 1983;95(3):359-363. doi:10.1016/S0002-9394(14)78306-0.

10. Lee GA, Hirst LW. Ocular surface squamous neoplasia. *Surv Ophthalmol.* 1995;39(6):429-450. doi:10.1016/S0039-6257(05)80054-2.

11. Hwang IP, Jordan DR, Brownstein S, Gilberg SM, McEachren TM, Prokopetz R. Mucoepidermoid carcinoma of the conjunctiva: a series of three cases. *Ophthalmology.* 2000; 107(4):801-805. doi:10.1016/S0161-6420(99)00177-3.

12. Rao NA, Font RL. Mucoepidermoid carcinoma of the conjunctiva: a clinicopathologic study of five cases. *Cancer.* 1976;38(4):1699-1709.

13. Chao AN, Shields CL, Krema H, Shields JA. Outcome of patients with periocular sebaceous gland carcinoma with and without conjunctival intraepithelial invasion. *Ophthalmology.* 2001;108(10):1877-1883. doi:10.1016/S0161-6420(01)00719-9.

14. Jakobiec FA. Sebaceous tumors of the ocular adnexa. In: Albert DM, Jakobiec FA, eds. *Principles and Practice of Ophthalmology.* Philadelphia, PA: WB Saunders; 1994.

15. Shields CL, Shields JA. Tumors of the conjunctiva and cornea. *Surv Ophthalmol.* 2004; 49(1):3-24. doi:10.1016/j.survophthal.2003.10.008.

16. Shields CL, Fasiuddin AF, Mashayekhi A, Shields JA. Conjunctival nevi: clinical features and natural course in 410 consecutive patients. *Arch Ophthalmol.* 2004;122(2):167-175. doi:10.1001/archopht.122.2.167.

17. Shields J, Shields CL, Mashayekhi A, et al. Primary acquired melanosis of the conjunctiva: risks for progression to melanoma in 311 eyes. The 2006 Lorenz E Zimmerman Lecture. *Ophthalmology.* 2008;115(3):511-519.e2. doi:10.1016/j.ophtha.2007.07.003.

18. Brownstein S, Jakobiec FA, Wilkinson RD, Lombardo J, Jackson WB. Cryotherapy for precancerous melanosis (atypical melanocytic hyperplasia) of the conjunctiva. *Arch Ophthalmol.* 1981;99(7):1224-1231. doi:10.1001/archopht.1981.03930020098009.

19. Fuchs U, Kivelä T, Liesto K, Tarkkanen A. Prognosis of conjunctival melanomas in relation to histological features. *Br J Cancer.* 1989;59(2):261-267.

20. Shields CL, Shields JA, Gündüz K, et al. Conjunctival melanoma: risk factors for recurrence, exenteration, metastasis and death in 150 consecutive patients. *Arch Ophthalmol.* 2000;118(11):1497-1507. doi:10.1001/archopht.118.11.1497.

21. Jakobiec FA. Corneal tumors. In: Kaufman HE, Barron BA, McDonald MB, Waltman SR, eds. *The Cornea.* New York, NY: Churchill Livingstone; 1988.

22. Ferry AP. Pyogenic granulomas of the eye and ocular adnexa: a study of 100 cases. *Trans Am Ophthalmol Soc.* 1989;87:327-343; discussion 343-347.

23. Howard G, Jakobiec FA, DeVoe AG. Kaposi's sarcoma of the conjunctiva. *Am J Ophthalmol.* 1975;79(3):420-423.

24. Weiter JJ, Jakobiec FA, Iwamoto T. The clinical and morphologic characteristics of Kaposi's sarcoma of the conjunctiva. *Am J Ophthalmol.* 1980;89(4):546-552. doi:10.1016/0002-9394(80)90064-1.

25. Goble RR, Frangoulis MA. Lymphangioma circumscriptum of the eyelids and conjunctiva. *Br J Ophthalmol.* 1990;74:574-575. doi:10.1136/bjo.74.9.574.

26. Ferry JA, Fung CY, Zukerberg L, et al. Lymphoma of the ocular adnexa: a study of 353 cases. *Am J Surg Pathol.* 2007;31(2):170-184. doi:10.1097/01.pas.0000213350.49767.46.

27. Knowles DM, Jakobiec FA, McNally L, Burke JS. Lymphoid hyperplasia and malignant lymphoma occurring in the ocular adnexa (orbit, conjunctiva, and eyelids): a prospective multiparametric analysis of 108 cases during 1977 to 1987. *Hum Pathol.* 1989;21(9):959-973.

28. Lachapelle KR. Treatment of conjunctival mucosa-associated lymphoid tissue lymphoma with intralesional interferon alpha-2b. *Arch Ophthalmol.* 2000;118:284.

8

Developmental Disorders

MICROCORNEA

Horizontal corneal diameter of < 9 mm in newborns or < 10 mm in adults. It is inherited in autosomal dominant or recessive manner and may be associated with systemic syndromes (Figure 8-1).

Signs and Symptoms. Small cornea, higher incidence of angle-closure glaucoma due to hyperopia. Other associated ocular findings include microphthalmos, anterior segment dysgenesis, congenital cataracts, persistent fetal vasculature, and optic nerve hypoplasia.

Exams and Tests. Measurement of horizontal corneal diameter, intraocular pressure, refraction, complete eye exam to evaluate for other ocular abnormalities, genetic testing.

Treatment. Managing refractive error, optimizing intraocular pressure, and managing other ocular abnormalities.

Kim T, Daluvoy MB.
The Pocket Guide to Cornea (pp 93-100).
© 2019 SLACK Incorporated.

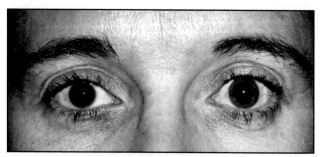

Figure 8-1. Microcornea. This external photo demonstrates asymmetry in corneal diameter, with microcornea of the right eye.

MEGALOCORNEA

Horizontal corneal diameter of > 12 mm in newborns or > 13 mm in adults. It is inherited in an X-linked fashion and may be associated with systemic syndromes.

Signs and Symptoms. Large but clear cornea, deep anterior chamber, normal intraocular pressure, high myopia. Other associated ocular findings include ectopia lentis, cataract, arcus juvenilis, and miosis.

Exams and Tests. Measurement of horizontal corneal diameter, rule out congenital glaucoma, complete eye exam to evaluate for other ocular abnormalities, genetic testing.

Treatment. Manage refractive error and other ocular abnormalities.

CORNEA PLANA

Congenital bilateral flat corneas with power less than 43 diopters. It is inherited in autosomal recessive or dominant manner and thought to be due to mutations in the KERA gene.

Signs and Symptoms. Decreased vision, hyperopia, shallow anterior chamber, glaucoma. Other associated ocular findings include aniridia, colobomas, anterior segment dysgenesis, and cataracts.

Exams and Tests. Measurement of corneal curvature, intraocular pressure, refraction, complete eye exam to assess for other ocular abnormalities, genetic testing.

Treatment. Manage refractive error, optimize glaucoma if present, manage other ocular abnormalities.

PETERS ANOMALY

Congenital abnormality caused by central absence of Descemet's membrane leading to central corneal opacity. Most cases are sporadic, but it can also be autosomal dominant or recessive. Most cases are bilateral.

Signs and Symptoms. Corneal clouding at birth, iridocorneal adhesions (type I), iridolental adhesions (type II), corectopia, shallow anterior chamber, glaucoma (Figure 8-2). Other associated ocular findings include aniridia, persistent fetal vasculature, cataract, ectopia lentis, microcornea. Systemic abnormalities (Peters plus syndrome) include cleft lip/palate, heart defects, central nervous system abnormalities, genitourinary or gastrointestinal malformations, skeletal dysplasia, and short stature.

Exams and Tests. Complete eye exam to assess for ocular abnormalities, intraocular pressure, genetic testing, evaluation for systemic findings.

Treatment. Optical iridectomy if the opacity is small enough to allow adequate light entry peripherally. If the opacity is too large to be amenable to management with optical iridectomy, early penetrating keratoplasty may be necessary to allow for development and maturation of the visual system. Management also involves surgical correction of pupillary abnormalities and control of intraocular pressure.

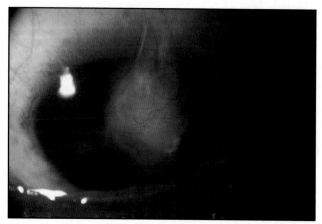

Figure 8-2. Peters anomaly. Corneal opacification associated with a focal absence of endothelium and Descemet's membrane and iridocorneal adhesions is seen. This image demonstrates associated corneal neovascularization.

SCLEROCORNEA

Congenital scleralization of the peripheral or entire cornea. It is sporadic but can also be transmitted in an autosomal dominant or recessive manner (Table 8-1).

Signs and Symptoms. Nonprogressive and noninflammatory scleralization and vascularization of the peripheral or entire cornea, cornea plana (Figure 8-3). Other associated ocular findings include anterior segment dysgenesis, glaucoma, and cataract.

Exams and Tests. Measurement of corneal curvature, intraocular pressure, refraction if subtotal scleralization, complete eye exam to assess for other ocular abnormalities.

Treatment. Penetrating keratoplasty (poor prognosis), manage other ocular abnormalities.

Table 8-1. Differential Diagnosis for Congenital Corneal Opacification

Birth trauma

Congenital glaucoma

Congenital hereditary endothelial dystrophy

Congenital hereditary stromal dystrophy

Corneal ulcer

Limbal dermoid

Metabolic

    Cystinosis

    Mucopolysaccharidoses

    Tyrosinemia

Peters anomaly

Sclerocornea

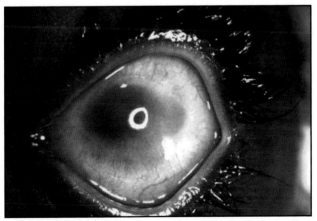

Figure 8-3. Sclerocornea. The peripheral cornea demonstrates an appearance more consistent with that of sclera.

AXENFELD-RIEGER SYNDROME

Bilateral anterior segment dysgenesis transmitted in an autosomal dominant manner.

Signs and Symptoms. Posterior embryotoxon (prominent and anteriorly displaced Schwalbe line), iris hypoplasia, corectopia, polycoria, glaucoma. Associated systemic findings include skeletal deformities, periumbilical abnormalities, hypospadias, pituitary dysfunction, cardiac defects, or deafness.

Exams and Tests. Complete eye exam to assess for other ocular abnormalities, intraocular pressure, genetic testing, evaluation for systemic abnormalities.

Treatment. Management of glaucoma, tinted contact lenses for photophobia, management of other ocular abnormalities.

CONGENITAL CORNEAL ANESTHESIA

Rare congenital hypoesthesia or anesthesia associated with trigeminal anesthesia, mesenchymal dysplasia, or hindbrain hypoplasia.

Signs and Symptoms. Blurry vision, recurrent painless corneal ulcerations, or corneal scarring.

Exams and Tests. Corneal sensation before administration of topical anesthetic, referral to pediatrician or geneticist to rule out systemic disorders.

Treatment. Aggressive lubrication, punctal occlusion, scleral contact lenses, tarsorrhaphy, amniotic membrane, or conjunctival flap in advanced cases.

EPIBULBAR DERMOID

A choristomatous growth of the epislcera typically found at the inferotemporal corneoscleral limbus (and therefore often referred to as limbal dermoids) and extending onto the surface of the cornea. Epibulbar dermoids are typically slow-growing or stationary, vascular, whitish, dome-shaped lesions that may induce local corneal flattening. The induced astigmatism may lead to refractive amblyopia due to anisometropia. Limbal dermoids are seen in Goldenhar syndrome, which commonly also involves preauricular skin tags, micrognathia, vertebral hypoplasia, and varying degrees of hearing loss.

Signs and Symptoms. Appearance of whitish, dome-shaped lesion at the corneoscleral limbus. May be bilateral or unilateral. Patients will occasionally complain of persistent irritation due to localized tear film disruption.

Exam and Tests. Slit-lamp examination is typically adequate to identify the lesion. Attention should be paid to the depth and degree of corneal involvement of the lesion, as these criteria can help guide surgical resection if undertaken. Cycloplegic refraction and topography (if the patient is able to cooperate) can be helpful in determining the risk of the patient for development of amblyopia.

Treatment. If the amount of induced astigmatism is small, these lesions can be observed and anisometropia treated with glasses. If the amount of induced astigmatism is significant and would not be adequately corrected with glasses, surgical excision of the lesion can be undertaken. Surgical excision may also be considered for lesions that demonstrate continued growth or cause persistent irritation. As these lesions sometimes extend to the posterior cornea, complete resection is not advisable. Rather, a lamellar keratectomy/sclerectomy or "shave" approach to match the height of surrounding tissue and avoid dellen formation is typically employed. Defects, if present after excision, can be filled with amniotic membrane or split-thickness corneal tissue.

BIBLIOGRAPHY

1. Bhandari R, Ferri S, Whittaker B, Liu M, Lazzaro DR. Peters anomaly: review of the literature. *Cornea*. 2011;30(8):939-944. doi:10.1097/ICO.0b013e31820156a9.

2. Mannis MJ, Holland EJ, eds. *Cornea*. 4th ed. Edinburgh, Scotland: Elsevier Inc; 2016.

3. Weisenthal RW. *2013-2014 Basic and Clinical Science Course Section 8: External Disease and Cornea*. San Francisco, CA: American Academy of Ophthalmology; 2014.

4. Shields MB, Buckley E, Klintworth GK, Thresher R. Axenfeld-Rieger syndrome. A spectrum of developmental disorders. *Surv Ophthalmol*. 1985;29(6):387-409. doi:10.1016/0039-6257(85)90205-X.

5. Pirouzian A, Holz H, Merrill K, Sudesh R, Karlen K. Surgical management of pediatric limbal dermoids with sutureless amniotic membrane transplantation and augmentation. *J Pediatr Ophthalmol Strabismus*. 2012;49(2):114-119. doi:10.3928/01913913-20110823-01.

9

Degenerations and Depositions

CONJUNCTIVA

Pinguecula

Interpalpebral conjunctival lesion that is typically yellow-white in appearance. It results from elastotic degeneration of subepithelial collagen (Figure 9-1).

Signs and Symptoms. Most commonly found nasally, can be highly vascularized or associated with adjacent punctate epithelial erosions or dellen due to abnormal tear film distribution. The lesions are typically asymptomatic but can become inflamed in some cases (pingueculitis).

Exams and Tests. Slit-lamp examination.

Treatment. Observation, lubrication, short courses of topical steroids or nonsteroidal anti-inflammatory drugs for inflammation. Though rare, cosmetically unacceptable pingueculae can be addressed by photocoagulation or surgical excision.

Kim T, Daluvoy MB.
The Pocket Guide to Cornea (pp 101-115).
© 2019 SLACK Incorporated.

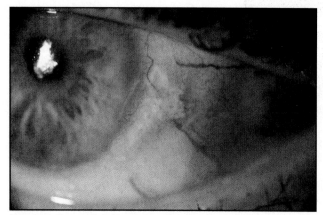

Figure 9-1. Pingueculum. The pingueculum seen in this image is a yellowish-white interpalpebral conjunctival lesion adjacent to the limbus.

Pterygium

A wing-shaped lesion of the interpalpebral conjunctiva that crosses the limbus onto the cornea, resulting from elastotic degeneration of subepithelial collagen.

Signs and Symptoms. Like pingueculae, pterygia are more commonly found nasally. Unlike pingueculae, pterygia are typically triangular, with the apex extending onto the corneal surface (Figure 9-2). They may also be associated with an iron line (Stocker line), indicating chronicity. They can cause dryness and ocular surface irritation, resulting from abnormal tear film distribution over the elevated lesion. They can appear injected and cause astigmatism.

Exams and Tests. Slit-lamp examination to measure its extension onto the cornea, fluorescein staining to evaluate for epithelial erosions and dellen. If the lesion is extensive, corneal topography can demonstrate flattening in the meridian of the lesion.

Treatment. Observation. If the lesion becomes cosmetically unacceptable, causes significant refractive change, or causes irritation, surgical excision can be undertaken. Excision is typically

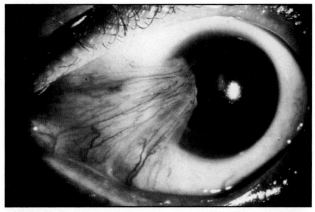

Figure 9-2. Pterygium. A wing-shaped conjunctival lesion is seen extending onto the corneal surface.

performed with amniotic membrane transplant or autologous conjunctival graft (lower rate of recurrence, 5% to 10%) with or without use of an antimetabolite such as mitomycin C.

Conjunctival Epithelial Inclusion Cyst

Benign fluid-filled lesion of the conjunctiva that is typically translucent and may be congenital or acquired (Figure 9-3).

Signs and Symptoms. Patients with conjunctival epithelial inclusion cysts are typically asymptomatic. They may note the cosmetic appearance of the lesion or begin to note ocular surface irritation due to tear film disruption or exposure.

Exams and Tests. Slit-lamp examination is typically sufficient. Histopathologic examination typically demonstrates a cavity lined by nonkeratinized epithelium with scattered goblet cells.

Treatment. If the patient is asymptomatic, no treatment is necessary. For patients who are symptomatic, excision of the inclusion cyst may be performed.

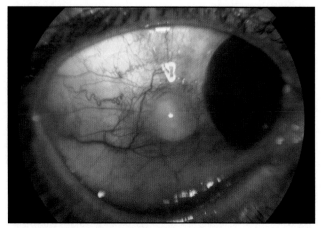

Figure 9-3. Conjunctival epithelial inclusion cyst. The cyst presents as a smooth, raised, translucent, fluid-filled lesion of the conjunctiva.

Conjunctivochalasis

Loose, redundant conjunctiva due to inflammation or age that can override the lower eyelid margin when severe (Figure 9-4).

Signs and Symptoms. Asymptomatic or can cause foreign body sensation, tearing (due to covering lower puncta), blurry vision, subconjunctival hemorrhages.

Exams and Tests. Slit-lamp examination is typically sufficient.

Treatment. Observation unless symptomatic, in which case it can be lasered, cauterized, or surgically removed.

CORNEA

Band Keratopathy

Calcium deposition within the corneal epithelial basement membrane, Bowman's layer, and anterior stroma (Figure 9-5).

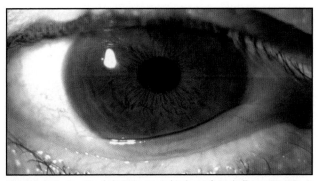

Figure 9-4. Conjunctivochalasis. Loose, redundant inferior bulbar conjunctiva is seen overlying the inferior cornea.

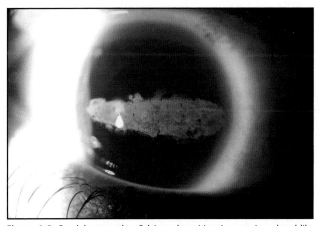

Figure 9-5. Band keratopathy. Calcium deposition is seen in a band-like interpalpebral distribution with limbal clear zones nasally and temporally.

Signs and Symptoms. Typically located in the interpalpebral anterior cornea with a clear interval separating the deposition from the corneal limbus. Subepithelial deposits of calcium are noted to coalesce over time, resulting in the typical horizontal "band" appearance. While chronic ocular inflammation and hypercalcemia are the 2 most common causes of band keratopathy, hyperphosphatemia (as may occur in renal failure), hereditary transmission, and silicone oil instillation (for retinal detachment management) are all known to be associated with band keratopathy.

Exam and Tests. Slit-lamp examination. If the patient has no known cause of chronic ocular inflammation, systemic evaluation for conditions may be warranted. Initial workup should include serum electrolytes and urinalysis.

Treatment. If band keratopathy becomes clinically significant (irritation or decreased vision), calcium chelation can be performed using ethylenediaminetetraacetic acid (EDTA) 0.5% to 1.5%. Epithelium is removed prior to applying the EDTA solution. If necessary, mild agitation or gentle scraping of the surface can be performed to enhance the removal of calcium. Manage any known systemic condition.

Iron Deposition

Brownish discoloration that occurs in the corneal epithelium as a result of chronic pooling of tears in particular regions of the cornea (Figure 9-6). This pooling is often related to elevations or depressions in or adjacent to the cornea.

Signs and Symptoms. Typically asymptomatic. Types of epithelial iron line locations include the superior border of the tear lake (Hudson-Stahli), the apex of a pterygium (Stocker), the border of a glaucoma-filtering bleb (Ferry), the cone in a keratoconic cornea (Fleischer), and anterior to keratoplasty sutures (Mannis). Iron may also be seen in the form of a "Coats white ring," which is a superficial deposition of iron that remains after removal of a metallic foreign body. Iron deposition in the posterior cornea may occur as the result of ocular siderosis due to a metallic intraocular foreign body or systemic iron overload.

Exams and Tests. Slit-lamp examination is typically sufficient. If the etiology of an anterior iron deposition is unclear, consider corneal topography to evaluate for abnormalities of corneal

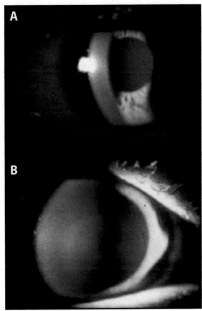

Figure 9-6. Iron lines. (A) Demonstrates an iron line within the slit beam. (B) Demonstrates an elliptical iron line.

shape. If posterior deposition is noted in the setting of a trauma history, dilated examination with or without computed tomography should be performed to rule out metallic intraocular foreign body. Systemic evaluation for iron overload should be performed if no intraocular cause of posterior iron deposition is noted.

Treatment. Treatment is not necessary. If associated with systemic iron overload, appropriate systemic management is indicated.

Corneal Arcus

A deposition of lipid in the peripheral cornea. It is thought to be related to the permeability of the limbal vasculature.

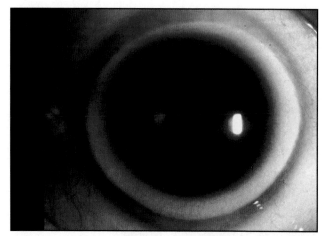

Figure 9-7. Corneal arcus. Image demonstrates whitish haze of the peripheral cornea with a small lucid interval at the corneoscleral limbus.

Signs and Symptoms. Arcus appears as a whitish, hazy deposition in the anterior and posterior portions of the peripheral cornea (Figure 9-7), with a small lucid interval between the deposition and the corneal limbus. Arcus occurs in 2 typical forms: in the elderly and in patients with dyslipidemia. Arcus in a young patient should raise the possibility of a disorder of lipid metabolism, such as familial hypercholesterolemia. Arcus that is highly asymmetric or unilateral (particularly in elderly patients) should raise the possibility of ocular ischemia (often related to asymmetric carotid disease) in the eye with little or no arcus.

Exams and Tests. Slit-lamp examination. If the patient is young, a lipid panel is warranted. In a patient with asymmetric arcus, carotid evaluation with Doppler ultrasound is warranted. In both populations, further evaluation by the patient's primary care provider is appropriate.

Treatment. Symmetric arcus in an elderly patient is observed. Management of any underlying condition as appropriate.

Senile Furrow Degeneration

A rare condition consisting of thinning occurring between the limbal vascular arcades and corneal arcus.

Signs and Symptoms. Typically asymptomatic, without associated changes in refraction. The thinning is not associated with vascularization or perforation but can be of relevance when planning anterior segment surgery.

Exams and Tests. Slit-lamp examination is sufficient to evaluate senile furrow degeneration.

Treatment. No treatment is indicated. If planning anterior segment surgery, areas of thinning should be noted, as corneal incisions through such areas may be structurally weaker and less likely to self-seal than incisions in a normal cornea.

Terrien Marginal Degeneration

A progressive, typically painless condition with characteristic peripheral stromal thinning of unknown etiology (Figure 9-8).

Signs and Symptoms. Typically a young patient (20 to 40 years of age) with progressive changes in refraction requiring frequent changes in glasses or contact lens correction. There is a 3:1 male predominance, with bilateral and symmetric thinning of the superior peripheral corneal stroma. Patients often demonstrate a yellow-white leading edge of lipid anterior to the area of thinning, punctate opacities in the anterior stroma, superficial vascularization from the limbal arcades, and an intact overlying epithelium. The thinning results in progressive against-the-rule astigmatism. Fifteen percent of patients will perforate spontaneously or with minor trauma.

Exams and Tests. Slit-lamp examination is often sufficient to confirm the diagnosis, with intact overlying epithelium, a leading edge of lipid, and the lack of association with pain or systemic inflammatory conditions differentiating the condition from other forms of peripheral corneal thinning (eg, Mooren's ulcer). Corneal topography and optical coherence tomography can

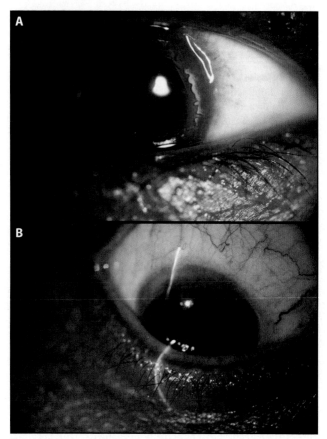

Figure 9-8. Terrien marginal degeneration. (A) Demonstrates peripheral corneal thinning with a leading edge of lipid. (B) Demonstrates peripheral corneal thinning confined to the classic superior distribution.

provide an indication of the extent of refractive change and corneal thinning, respectively.

Treatment. Refractive changes can be managed with glasses or contact lenses. No treatment exists to prevent the progression of thinning. If thinning is severe, a crescentic lamellar or eccentric penetrating graft can be used to stabilize the affected area of the cornea.

Salzmann Nodular Degeneration

Slowly progressive condition of elevated white nodules near the limbus or in midperiphery (Figure 9-9). The etiology is unknown but may be related to prior corneal inflammation.

Signs and Symptoms. Typically asymptomatic, but may present with dry eye or ocular surface irritation due to tear film irregularity. Nodules that are in the visual axis may result in decreased vision.

Exams and Tests. Slit-lamp examination and corneal topography can be used to evaluate changes associated with Salzmann nodules.

Treatment. Observation. Ocular irritation can be managed with lubrication. Nodules in the visual axis or causing significant tear film irregularity may be managed with superficial keratectomy and/or phototherapeutic keratectomy.

Cornea Verticillata

A whorl-like pattern of mild epithelial opacities that can result from systemic conditions such as the X-linked lysosomal storage disorder Fabry disease or usage of a variety of medications, including amiodarone, chloroquine, chlorpromazine, indomethacin, and naproxen (Figure 9-10).

Signs and Symptoms. Typically asymptomatic and usually presents as an incidental finding on ophthalmic examination. Deposits may vary from brown to white in color. The superficial deposition indicates likely secretion of deposited materials or medications in the tear film.

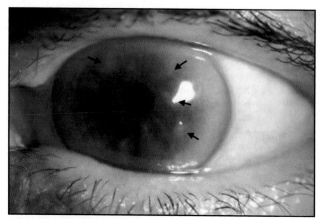

Figure 9-9. Salzmann nodular degeneration. Multiple whitish nodular elevations are seen on the corneal surface (arrows).

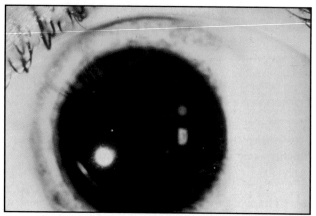

Figure 9-10. Cornea verticillata. A whorl-like pattern of corneal epithelial opacification is seen.

Exams and Tests. Slit-lamp examination is sufficient. Any young patient with a family history of Fabry disease should be evaluated further by his or her primary care provider.

Treatment. No treatment needed. Management of Fabry disease (and possibly genetic counseling for possible carriers of Fabry disease) is warranted for affected patients.

Iridocorneal Endothelial Syndrome

A unilateral, nonfamilial disorder with typical onset in young adulthood involving abnormalities of the corneal endothelium and iris. There are 3 forms of iridocorneal endothelial (ICE) syndrome (iris nevus syndrome, Chandler syndrome, and essential iris atrophy), all of which involve an abnormally proliferating endothelium that lays down basement membrane across the anterior chamber angle and iris. Although a viral association has been suggested, no definitive evidence exists indicating the etiology of ICE syndrome.

Signs and Symptoms. Onset of symptoms is typically in young adulthood, more often in women than in men. Typical presenting symptoms include mild blurring of vision and a noticeable change in the iris. Endothelial dysfunction can lead to corneal edema, while membrane formation over the iris can lead to iris atrophy, corectopia, and polycoria. Glaucoma secondary to membrane formation over the anterior chamber angle is also common. As indicated by its name, essential iris atrophy predominantly involves varying degrees of iris atrophy, corectopia, and polycoria. The onset of Chandler syndrome is typically heralded by blurry vision and colored halos around lights as a result of corneal edema. Iris nevus syndrome involves a unilateral diffuse nevus of the iris, a matted iris appearance, and iris heterochromia.

Exams and Tests. Slit-lamp examination with specular reflection can reveal a "hammered silver" appearance of the corneal endothelium. Patchy iris atrophy, corectopia, polycoria, ectropion uveae, and unilateral diffuse nevus (in iris nevus syndrome) may be seen. Gonioscopy can reveal peripheral anterior synechiae. Specular microscopy can demonstrate dark/light reversal of the corneal endothelial cells (normally dark cell borders appear brighter than cellular contents on specular microscopy). Tonometry often reveals asymmetric elevation in intraocular pressure (IOP) in the affected eye.

Treatment. No treatment exists that directly addresses the progressive proliferation of abnormal endothelium involved in ICE syndrome. As a result, treatment focuses on addressing the glaucoma, corneal edema, and iris defects resulting from the condition. Treatment of glaucoma typically requires glaucoma-filtering surgery or glaucoma-drainage device implantation. Corneal edema can be managed early in the course with control of IOP and topical hypertonic solutions. Progressive corneal edema may require endothelial or penetrating keratoplasty. Treatment of iris defects is often poorly amenable to suture-based repair, and symptoms of glare and photophobia can in some cases be addressed with iris prostheses where available.

BIBLIOGRAPHY

1. Austin P, Jakobiec FA, Iwamoto T. Elastodysplasia and elastodystrophy as the pathologic basis of pterygia and pinguecula. *Ophthalmology.* 1983;90:96.
2. Boynton JR, Searl SS, Ferry AP, Kaltreider SA, Rodenhouse TG. Primary nonkeratinized epithelial ('conjunctival') orbital cysts. *Arch Ophthalmol.* 1992;110(9):1238-1242. doi:10.1001/archopht.1992.01080210056024.
3. Shields JA, Shields CL. Orbital cysts of childhood—classification, clinical features, and management. *Surv Ophthalmol.* 2004;49(3):281-299. doi:10.1016/j.survophthal.2004.02.001.
4. Vishwanath MR, Jain A. Conjunctival inclusion cyst following sub-Tenon's local anaesthetic injection. *Br J Anaesth.* 2005;95(6):825-826.
5. Cursino JW, Fine BS. A histologic study of calcific and noncalcific band keratopathies. *Am J Ophthalmol.* 1976;82(3):395-404.
6. Doughman DJ, Olson GA, Nolan S, Hajny RG. Experimental band keratopathy. *Arch Ophthalmol.* 1969;81(2):264-271.
7. Lemp MA, Ralph RA. Rapid development of band keratopathy in dry eyes. *Am J Ophthalmol.* 1977;83(5):657-659.
8. Wood TO, Walker GG. Treatment of band keratopathy. *Am J Ophthalmol.* 1975;80(3 Pt 2):550.

9. Rose GE, Lavin MJ. The Hudson-Stahli line. III: Observations on morphology, a critical review of aetiology and a unified theory for the formation of iron lines of the corneal epithelium. *Eye (Lond)*. 1987;1(Pt 4):475-479.

10. Barraquer-Somers E, Chan CC, Green WR. Corneal epithelial iron deposition. *Ophthalmology*. 1983;90(6):729-734.

11. Cogan DG, Kuwabara T. Arcus senilis: its pathology and histochemistry. *AMA Arch Ophthalmol*. 1959;61(4):553-560.

12. Rifkind BM. Corneal arcus and hyperlipoproteinemia. *Surv Ophthalmol*. 1972;16(5):295-304.

13. Sugar A. Corneal and conjunctival degenerations. In: Kaufman HE, Barron BA, McDonald MB, Waltman SR, eds. *The Cornea*. New York, NY: Churchill Livingstone; 1988.

14. Beauchamp GR. Terrien's marginal corneal degeneration. *J Pediatr Ophthalmol Strabismus*. 1982;19(2):97-99.

15. Austin P, Brown SI. Inflammatory Terrien's marginal corneal disease. *Am J Ophthalmol*. 1981;92(2):189-192.

16. Wood TO. Salzmann's nodular degeneration. *Cornea*. 1990;9(1):17-22.

17. Farjo AA, Halperin GI, Syed N, Sutphin JE, Wagoner MD. Salzmann's nodular corneal degeneration clinical characteristics and surgical outcomes. *Cornea*. 2006;25(1):11-15.

18. Kaplan LJ, Cappaert WE. Amiodarone keratopathy. Correlation to dosage and duration. *Arch Ophthalmol*. 1982;100(4):601-602.

19. Johnson AW, Buffaloe WJ. Chlorpromazine epithelial keratopathy. *Arch Ophthalmol*. 1966;76(5):664-667.

20. Sher NA, Letson RD, Desnick RJ. The ocular manifestations in Fabry's disease. *Arch Ophthalmol*. 1979;97(4):671-676.

10

Corneal Dystrophies

EPITHELIAL AND SUBEPITHELIAL

Epithelial Basement Membrane Dystrophy

EBMD is the most common anterior corneal dystrophy. It is characterized by microcystic changes, map-like gray areas with intervening clear zones, and "fingerprint" lines within the corneal epithelium.

Signs and Symptoms. Asymptomatic or present with blurred vision, irritation, and recurrent corneal erosions. Patients commonly describe pain when opening their eyes upon awakening, due to erosion occurring in the setting of traction on the epithelial surface from the eyelids. Pain ranges from a few minutes to a few days, depending on the severity of the erosion.

Exams and Tests. Slit-lamp examination is typically sufficient to diagnose EBMD. Fluorescein staining may be helpful to identify areas of negative staining and retroillumination can highlight area of irregularity (Figure 10-1).

Kim T, Daluvoy MB.
The Pocket Guide to Cornea (pp 117-138).
© 2019 SLACK Incorporated.

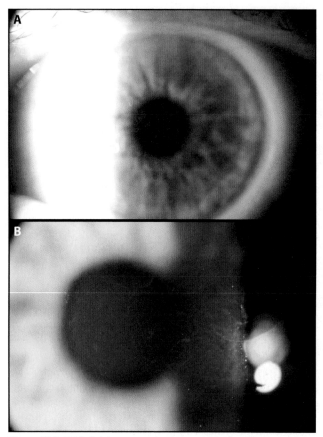

Figure 10-1. Epithelial basement membrane dystrophy. (A) Demonstrates fingerprint lines. (B) Demonstrates map lines.

Treatment. Management is aimed at addressing decreased vision and recurrent corneal erosion. Lubrication can reduce traction on the corneal epithelium, while hypertonic solutions and ointments (particular when applied before sleep) can limit development of

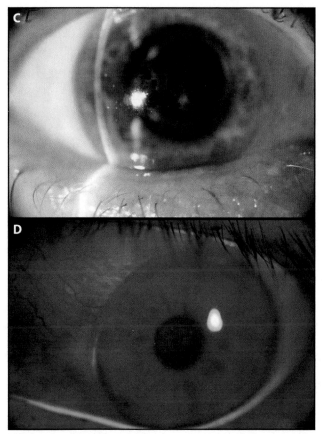

Figure 10-1 (continued). (C) Demonstrates epithelial microcysts and corneal erosion. (D) Demonstrates highlighting of map lines with the use of fluorescein.

epithelial edema and may improve epithelial adhesion. Bandage contact lenses may also be used for short periods. More severe erosions may be treated with epithelial debridement, diamond burr polishing, anterior stromal micropuncture. Phototherapeutic

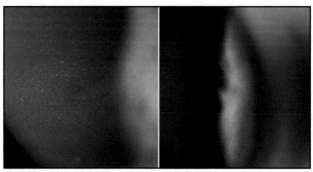

Figure 10-2. Meesmann epithelial corneal dystrophy. Epithelial microcysts are seen. (Reprinted with permission from Dr. Ramon Coral Ghanem.)

keratectomy (PTK) using an excimer laser may provide more lasting therapy.

Meesmann Epithelial Corneal Dystrophy

MECD is a clinically mild dystrophy related to mutation in corneal keratin and associated with intraepithelial microcysts containing degenerated epithelial cells.

Signs and Symptoms. Patients are typically asymptomatic; microcysts can be seen best on retroillumination. Small-scale erosions may occasionally occur (Figure 10-2).

Exams and Tests. Slit-lamp examination with retroillumination is helpful in identifying this dystrophy. Epithelial cells in patients with MECD are described on electron microscopy as containing granular or filamentary material referred to as "peculiar substance."

Inheritance. Autosomal dominant.

Genetic Associations. Keratin genes K3 and K12.

Treatment. Lubrication is generally sufficient because of the mild nature of the condition.

Lisch Epithelial Corneal Dystrophy

LECD is characterized by whorl- and band-shaped epithelial microcysts.

Signs and Symptoms. Patients are typically asymptomatic, but may note blurring of vision if the central cornea is involved.

Exams and Tests. Slit-lamp examination is sufficient for identification of this condition.

Treatment. Lubrication is typically sufficient.

Gelatinous Droplike Corneal Dystrophy

Also known as GDCD, involves subepithelial and stromal deposits of amyloid.

Signs and Symptoms. Patients often become symptomatic within the first or second decade of life, demonstrating 1 of 3 typical patterns: mulberry, band keratopathy, or kumquat. The mulberry type involves formation of nodular clusters, while the band keratopathy type involves a grayish-whitish band of subepithelial opacification. The kumquat type of GDCD involves yellowish stromal opacification throughout the cornea. Patients reports substantial photophobia, irritation, and decreased vision.

Exams and Tests. Slit-lamp examination is sufficient for identification of this condition. Histopathologic examination demonstrates basal epithelial, subepithelial, and stromal deposits of amyloid.

Inheritance. Autosomal recessive.

Genetic Association. TACSTD2 (1p32).

Treatment. Epithelial erosions can be managed with lubrication and bandage contact lenses. As deposition worsens superficial keratectomy, lamellar keratoplasty, or penetrating keratoplasty (PK) may be undertaken. However, GDCD typically recurs within grafts.

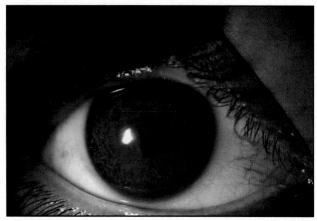

Figure 10-3. Reis-Bücklers corneal dystrophy. The image depicts mottled subepithelial clouding.

Bowman's Layer

Reis-Bücklers Corneal Dystrophy

RBCD is an early, progressive clouding of the cornea due to degenerative changes in the deep epithelium and Bowman's layer.

Signs and Symptoms. Normal corneas at birth develop progressive subepithelial deposition leading to blurred vision and recurrent erosions within the first decade of life (Figure 10-3).

Exams and Tests. Slit-lamp examination is sufficient to identify this condition. Masson trichrome and electron microscopy can aid in confirmation of the diagnosis and differentiation from Thiel-Behnke corneal dystrophy (TBCD) (see the following).

Inheritance. Autosomal dominant.

Genetic Association. TGFB1 (5q).

Treatment. Early in the disease, therapy may consist of lubrication with or without bandage contact lens. As deposition worsens and erosions become more frequent, PTK with or without topical mitomycin C becomes the treatment of choice. PTK can be repeated if deposition recurs, which is common. As deposition becomes deeper, deep anterior lamellar keratoplasty or PK may be indicated. However, recurrence of the dystrophy in grafts is common.

Thiel-Behnke Corneal Dystrophy

TBCD is a dystrophy of the Bowman's layer similar in appearance to RBCD. TBCD is also referred to as honeycomb-shaped corneal dystrophy because of its appearance on slit-lamp examination.

Signs and Symptoms. Normal corneas at birth develop honeycomb-shaped changes in the Bowman's layer within the first and second decades of life. Recurrent erosions can begin in childhood, with decreased vision occurring later.

Exams and Tests. Slit-lamp examination is sufficient to identify this condition. Electron microscopy can aid in confirmation of the diagnosis and differentiation from RBCD by the presence of "curly fibers" in TBCD and "rod-shaped bodies" in RBCD. In addition, Masson trichrome stains TBCD only weakly, as opposed to strong staining in RBCD.

Inheritance. Autosomal dominant.

Genetic Association. TGFBI (10q24).

Treatment. Management is similar to that of RBCD, with early treatment involving lubrication and therapy for corneal erosions. PTK is the treatment of choice for visually significant deposition or frequent erosions. Deep anterior lamellar keratoplasty or PK may be indicated for deeper deposition, but recurrence is common.

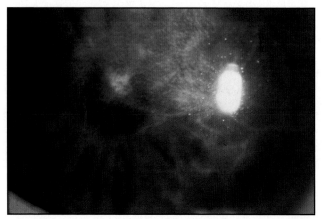

Figure 10-4. Lattice corneal dystrophy. Amyloid deposition is seen in the form of fine refractile lines in anterior stroma.

STROMAL

Transforming Growth Factor-Beta Induced

Lattice Corneal Dystrophy. LCD is a Transforming Growth Factor-Beta Induced (TGFBI) corneal dystrophy with 2 subtypes: the classic form (LCD1) and the gelsolin type (LCD2). LCD1 is a bilateral amyloidosis localized to the cornea. LCD2 (also called Meretoja syndrome) is a systemic amyloidosis affecting several organ systems associated with corneal amyloid deposition. Owing to the systemic nature of LCD2, it is not a true corneal dystrophy.

Signs and Symptoms. Patients with LCD1 typically have onset of findings within the first decade of life, beginning with anterior stromal white dots progressing to include fine refractile lines with diffuse anterior and mid stromal haze (Figure 10-4). The periphery of the cornea is typically clear. Amyloid deposition results in poor visual acuity by 40 years of age, and corneal erosions are frequent.

Patients with LCD2 typically have good vision through the first 6 decades of life. The refractile lines are thicker and more peripheral than those found in LCD1 and corneal erosions are rare. These patients have amyloidosis that results in facial paresis, laxity of facial skin, and cardiac conduction abnormalities.

Exams and Tests. Slit-lamp examination is typically sufficient to diagnose LCD. The presence or absence of systemic findings such as facial paresis and skin laxity can aid in the differentiation between LCD1 and LCD2. Histopathologic examination reveals orange-red staining of fusiform amyloid deposits with Congo red. Deposits stained with Congo red demonstrate apple-green birefringence when viewed with polarized light. Deposits demonstrate metachromasia when stained with crystal violet.

Inheritance. Autosomal dominant.

Genetic Associations. LCD1: TGFBI (5q31); LCD2: Gelsolin gene, GSN (9q34).

Treatment. Recurrent erosions are treated with lubrication and bandage contact lenses. PTK can be used for superficial opacification. Involvement of midstroma may require lamellar or PK. LCD recurs in grafts more commonly than macular and granular dystrophies.

Granular Dystrophy.
A TGFBI corneal dystrophy with 3 subtypes: the classic type (GCD1), the combined granular-lattice type (GCD2, also called Avellino corneal dystrophy), and the anterior form (RBCD; see previous section). This section pertains specifically to GCD1.

Signs and Symptoms. GCD1 is characterized by crumb-like, grayish-white opacifications in the anterior and midstroma with intervening clear spaces (Figure 10-5). After the fifth decade of life, opacification of the intervening stroma can occur, leading to decreased vision. Corneal erosions are common and photophobia may be present.

Exams and Tests. Slit-lamp examination is typically sufficient to identify GCD1. Histopathologic examination demonstrates bright red staining of hyaline deposits with Masson trichrome

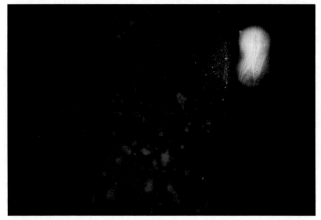

Figure 10-5. Granular corneal dystrophy. Crumb-like gray-white opacities are seen in anterior stroma.

stain. Electron microscopy demonstrates dense amorphous deposits with intervening microfibrils. Confocal microscopy demonstrates hyperreflective opacities within the stroma.

Inheritance. Autosomal dominant.

Genetic Association. TGFBI (5q31).

Treatment. Epithelial erosions can be managed with lubrication and bandage contact lenses. Opacification is rarely visually significant. If superficial, superficial keratectomy or PTK can be performed. Deeper lesions can be treated with lamellar or PK; however, GCD1 typically does not require surgical intervention. GCD1 can recur in grafts.

Avellino Corneal Dystrophy. GCD2 is a subtype of granular corneal dystrophy (see the previous example) referred to as GCD2. It demonstrates features both of granular dystrophy and lattice dystrophy.

Signs and Symptoms. Characterized by anterior stromal grayish-white granular opacities, posterior stromal refractile lines, and anterior stromal haze. The granular features typically develop first, followed by lattice features and finally haze. Corneal erosions are common.

Exams and Tests. Slit-lamp examination is typically sufficient to identify GCD2. Histopathologic examination demonstrates staining both with Masson trichrome and Congo red stains. Electron microscopy demonstrates features both of GCD1 and LCD.

Inheritance. Autosomal dominant.

Genetic Association. TGFBI (5q31).

Treatment. Management is similar to that for GCD1 and LCD. Epithelial erosions can be managed with lubrication and bandage contact lenses. Superficial opacification can be managed with superficial keratectomy or PTK. Deeper lesions can be treated with lamellar or PK. Recurrence in grafts can occur after keratoplasty.

Nontransforming Growth Factor-Beta Induced

Macular Corneal Dystrophy. MCD is characterized by stromal deposition of mucopolysaccharide.

Signs and Symptoms. Corneal changes are noted within the first decade of life, showing a ground-glass appearance of the central stroma that extends peripherally as the condition progresses (Figure 10-6). By the third decade, vision is often severely affected. Its course is punctuated by attacks involving irritation and photophobia.

Exams and Tests. Slit-lamp examination is typically sufficient to identify this condition, although it can appear similar to granular dystrophy in its early stages. Histopathologic examination demonstrates accumulation of glycosaminoglycans that stain with Alcian blue and colloidal iron. Electron microscopy demonstrates mucopolysaccharide accumulation within keratocytes.

Inheritance. Autosomal recessive.

Genetic Association. CHST6 gene (16q22).

Treatment. Photophobia can be managed with tinted contact lenses. Epithelial erosions can be managed with lubrication and bandage contact lenses. Superficial opacification can be managed

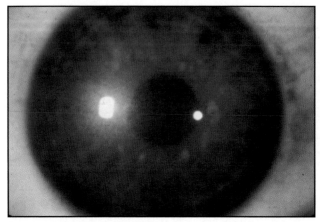

Figure 10-6. Macular corneal dystrophy. The stroma demonstrates a ground-glass appearance.

with superficial keratectomy or PTK. Deeper lesions can be treated with lamellar or PK. Recurrence in grafts can occur after keratoplasty.

Schnyder Crystalline Dystrophy.
SCD is a stromal dystrophy characterized by disc-shaped opacities consisting of fine cholesterol crystals (Figure 10-7).

Signs and Symptoms. Onset of findings in childhood. By the fourth decade, a diffuse stromal haze is typically present and corneal sensation may be decreased. This condition is associated with hypercholesterolemia, but the severity of disease does not correlate with severity of hypercholesterolemia. Thus, it likely represents a localized defect in lipid metabolism.

Exams and Tests. Slit-lamp examination is typically sufficient to identify this condition. Histopathologic examination demonstrates staining of deposited lipids with oil red O. There may also be focal or complete destruction of the Bowman's layer. Lipid panel is warranted to evaluate for hyperlipidemia.

Inheritance. Autosomal dominant.

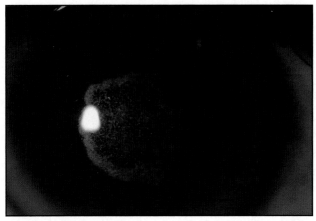

Figure 10-7. Schynder crystalline dystrophy. A disc-shaped central area with fine cholesterol crystals is seen.

Genetic Association. UBIAD1 (1p36).

Treatment. Early stages of disease have mild visual impairment, but later stages may require lamellar or PK. Cholesterol crystals may recur in grafts.

Congenital Stromal Corneal Dystrophy.

CSCD is a rare dystrophy that presents at birth with bilateral corneal haze with snowflake-like opacities. The condition is thought to be the result of disordered stromal fibrogenesis.

Signs and Symptoms. The presence of corneal clouding at birth can lead to deprivation amblyopia and sensory nystagmus. Epithelial erosions are rare.

Exams and Tests. Slit-lamp examination will demonstrate corneal clouding. Histopathologic examination demonstrates stromal regions with randomly oriented collagen fibrils. Collagen fibrils throughout the stroma are found to be abnormally small.

Inheritance. Autosomal dominant.

Genetic Association. DCN (12q21.33).

Treatment. Owing to concern for deprivation amblyopia, early PK is often indicated. While CSCD does not recur in grafts, visually acuity better than 20/200 is rarely achieved.

Fleck Corneal Dystrophy. FCD is a mild dystrophy involving faint, flat, grayish-whitish depositions throughout the stroma.

Signs and Symptoms. Identification is generally incidental during careful slit-lamp examination of the cornea as it is rarely symptomatic.

Exams and Tests. Slit-lamp examination is typically sufficient to identify this condition. Histopathologic examination demonstrates scattered abnormal keratocytes with excess glycosaminoglycan and lipid. These depositions stain with Alcian blue and oil red O, respectively.

Inheritance. Autosomal dominant.

Genetic Association. PIP5K3 (2q35).

Treatment. In general, no treatment is required as patients are asymptomatic.

Pre-Descemet Corneal Dystrophy. PDCD is characterized by fine gray punctate opacities in the posterior stroma.

Signs and Symptoms. Findings are typically seen incidentally after the third decade of life. Patients will generally have normal visual acuity.

Exams and Tests. Slit-lamp examination is typically sufficient to identify this condition. Histopathologic examination demonstrates abnormal keratocytes containing period acid-Schiff-positive material and lipid.

Inheritance. Unknown.

Genetic Association. Unknown.

Treatment. As patients are typically asymptomatic, no treatment is required.

Descemet Membrane and Endothelial

Fuchs' Endothelial Dystrophy. FECD is a slowly progressive condition characterized by corneal guttae, endothelial cell dysfunction, and corneal edema.

Signs and Symptoms. Typically noted in the fifth decade of life with central corneal guttae. Patients are typically asymptomatic in the early stages of the condition. As the condition slowly progresses, guttae may spread peripherally while Descemet membrane thickens and takes on a beaten-metal appearance. Patients commonly describe a variable blurring of the vision that is worse in the morning. Endothelial dysfunction in the setting of an abnormal Descemet membrane leads to corneal edema, progressing from posterior (stromal edema) to anterior (microcystic epithelial edema and bullae). Stromal opacification and subepithelial fibrosis can occur in the late stages of the condition.

An early-onset form of the condition also exists, with guttae presenting in the first decade of life. Guttae may be smaller than in the late-onset form. The early-onset form is slowly progressive, like the late-onset form, but because of its earlier onset, corneal decompensation occurs earlier in life.

Exams and Tests. Slit-lamp examination is typically sufficient to identify this condition. Retrocorneal illumination shows guttae well (Figure 10-8). Corneal pachymetry can be used to establish a baseline as well as track progression of corneal edema. Specular microscopy can highlight guttae as well as endothelial cell pleomorphism, polymegathism, and density reduction. These findings can also be noted on confocal microscopy. Histopathologic examination demonstrates thickened Descemet membrane with droplike excrescences surrounded by fibrous tissue, as well as reduction in endothelial cell density.

Inheritance. Autosomal dominant in some families, otherwise no clear inheritance pattern.

Genetic Associations. Classic FECD: possible SLC4A11; early-onset FECD: COL8A2 (1p34.3 to p32.3; L450W and Q455K mutations).

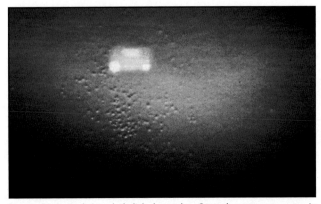

Figure 10-8. Fuchs' endothelial dystrophy. Corneal guttae are seen in retroillumination.

Treatment. In the early stages of FECD, patients are often asymptomatic. Hypertonic saline drops can help with early symptoms of the disease such as mild edema and morning blurring of vision. Corneal transplantation in various forms is considered the definitive treatment for FECD, as recurrence of FECD in grafts is not known to occur. While PK was commonly performed in the past, forms of posterior lamellar keratoplasty such as Descemet-stripping endothelial keratoplasty (DSEK) and Descemet membrane endothelial keratoplasty (DMEK) are routinely performed as they allow for faster visual recovery, greater structural integrity, decreased astigmatism, and better long-term visual acuity. While more data exist regarding the long-term outcomes of DSEK than DMEK, both procedures have demonstrated excellent rates of corneal clearing and graft survival thus far.

Posterior Polymorphous Corneal Dystrophy

PPCD is a highly variable condition characterized by "snail-track" and vesicular lesions at the level of the Descemet

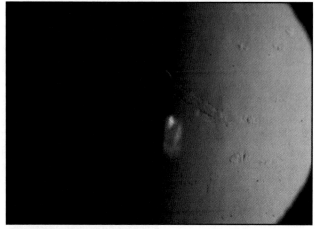

Figure 10-9. Posterior polymorphous dystrophy. "Snail tracks" are seen within Descemet membrane.

membrane with endothelial cells appearing and proliferating in a manner similar to that of epithelium (Figure 10 9).

Signs and Symptoms. Typically noted in the second or third decade of life as an incidental finding on routine examination. In some cases, however, it has an aggressive course that can manifest with decreased vision, corneal decompensation, and glaucoma. Three typical lesions are seen: vesicular lesions, "snail-track" lesions with scalloped borders, and diffuse opacities at the level of the Descemet membrane. Peripheral anterior synechiae can also be seen, resulting from migration of abnormal endothelial cells across the trabecular meshwork.

Exams and Tests. Slit-lamp examination is typically sufficient to identify this condition. Monitoring for glaucoma is warranted. Histopathologic examination demonstrates patches of abnormal flattened, layered endothelial cells.

Inheritance. Autosomal dominant.

Figure 10-10. Congenital hereditary endothelial dystrophy. Corneal clouding and thickening are seen.

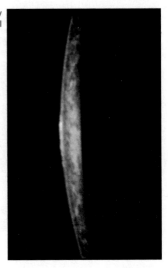

Genetic Associations. PPCD1 to unknown gene (20p11.2 to q11.2), PPCD2 to COL8A2 (1p34.3 to p32.3), PPCD3 to ZEB1 (10p11.2).

Treatment. PPCD is asymptomatic in most patients. In patients exhibiting aggressive disease, glaucoma should be treated appropriately. Rarely, corneal clouding requires PK. PPCD can recur after keratoplasty with the development of retrocorneal membranes that may be refractory to existing treatments.

Congenital Hereditary Endothelial Dystrophy 1

CHED1 is a rare condition characterized by corneal clouding developing after birth (typically around 9 to 15 months of age) that remains stable or slowly progressive (Figure 10-10).

Signs and Symptoms. Photophobia and epiphora often occur prior to onset of corneal clouding and may be the presenting symptoms. Corneal clouding and corneal thickening tend to occur toward the end of the first year of life. Visual acuity is typically 20/60 to 20/400 long term and patients typically do not develop nystagmus.

Exam and Tests. Complete ocular examination is necessary to diagnose this condition. Corneal pachymetry (elevated in CHED1) can be helpful in differentiating this condition from other causes of corneal clouding in infancy, such as mucopolysaccharidoses (normal pachymetry). Differentiation from glaucoma is also necessary, particularly given the onset of epiphora and photophobia prior to corneal clouding. Accordingly, intraocular pressure (IOP) testing is necessary. Histopathologic examination demonstrates areas of reduced, degenerated, or absent endothelial cells. Stromal thickness is often 2 to 3 times normal with a disrupted lamellar pattern, and some cases demonstrate subepithelial fibrosis and calcification.

Inheritance. Autosomal dominant.

Genetic Association. Unknown gene (20p11.2 to q11.2).

Treatment. Opacification can be managed with PK, but given the general stability of corneal clouding after onset, it may be delayed or avoided because of greater complication risk of PK in children. Endothelial keratoplasty has become the treatment of choice for these children, providing a lower risk option than PK for visual rehabilitation.

Congenital Hereditary Endothelial Dystrophy 2

CHED2 is a rare corneal dystrophy characterized by corneal clouding at birth due to areas of abnormality or absence of endothelial cells.

Signs and Symptoms. Patients typically demonstrate a grayish-bluish haze of the corneal stroma within the first week to 6 months of life. Owing to the early onset of corneal clouding, nystagmus is often present.

Exam and Tests. Complete ocular examination is necessary to diagnose this condition. Patients typically demonstrate significant thickening of the cornea on pachymetry. Differentiation from glaucoma is important. Accordingly, IOP testing is necessary.

Histopathologic examination demonstrates areas of reduced, degenerated, or absent endothelial cells. Stromal thickness is often 2 to 3 times normal with a disrupted lamellar pattern, and some cases demonstrate subepithelial fibrosis and calcification.

Inheritance. Autosomal recessive.

Genetic Association. SLC4A11 (20p13).

Treatment. Opacification can be managed with PK. Owing to the onset of clouding at birth, PK is often undertaken within the first 2 to 3 years. Accordingly, there is a low rate of graft survival and high rates of adverse effects, such as cataract and glaucoma. Endothelial keratoplasty may provide benefit in these children, despite the stromal disorganization, but data remain limited on this intervention for CHED2 at present.

BIBLIOGRAPHY

1. Cogan DG, Donaldson DD, Kuwabara T, Marshall D. Microcystic dystrophy of the corneal epithelium. *Trans Am Ophthalmol Soc.* 1964;63:213-225.
2. Cogan DG, Kuwabara T, Donaldson DD, Collins E. Microscopic dystrophy of the cornea. A partial explanation for its pathogenesis. *Arch Ophthalmol.* 1974;92(6):470-474.
3. Guerry DuP. Fingerprint-like lines in the cornea. *Am J Ophthalmol.* 1950;33(5):724-726.
4. Burns RP. Meesmann's corneal dystrophy. *Trans Am Ophthalmol Soc.* 1968;66:530-636.
5. Kuwabara T, Ciccarelli EC. Meesmann's corneal dystrophy. A pathological study. *Arch Ophthalmol.* 1964;71(5):676-682. doi:10.1001/archopht.1964.00970010692015.
6. Lisch WB, Büttner A, Offner F, et al. Lisch corneal dystrophy is genetically distinct from Meesmann corneal dystrophy and maps to xp22.3. *Am J Ophthalmol.* 2000;130(4):461-468.
7. Akiya S, Ito I, Matsui M. Gelatinous drop-like dystrophy of the cornea: light and electron microscopic study of superficial stromal lesion. *Jpn J Clin Ophthalmol.* 1972;26:815.
8. Weber FL, Babel J. Gelatinous drop-like dystrophy. *Arch Ophthalmol.* 1980;98(1):144-148.

9. Küchle M, Green WR, Volcker HE, Barraquer J. Reevaluation of corneal dystrophies of Bowman's layer and the anterior stroma (Reis-Bücklers' and Thiel-Behnke types): a light and electron microscopic study of eight corneas and a review of the literature. *Cornea*. 1995;14(4):333-354.

10. Perry HD, Fine BS, Caldwell DR. Reis-Bücklers' dystrophy. A study of eight cases. *Arch Ophthalmol*. 1979;97(4):664-670.

11. Dubord PJ, Krachmer JH. Diagnosis of early lattice corneal dystrophy. *Arch Ophthalmol*. 1982;100(5):788-790.

12. François J, Fehér J. Light microscopy and polarization optical study of the lattice dystrophy of the cornea. *Ophthalmologica*. 1972;164(1):1-18.

13. Bowen RA, Hassard DT, Wong VG, DeLellis RA, Glenner GG. Lattice dystrophy of the cornea as a variety of amyloidosis. *Am J Ophthalmol*. 1970;70(5):822-825.

14. Akiya S, Brown SI. Granular dystrophy of the cornea. Characteristic electron microscopic lesion. *Arch Ophthalmol*. 1970;84(2):179-192.

15. Sornson ET. Granular dystrophy of the cornea. An electron microscopic study. *Am J Ophthalmol*. 1965;59:1001-1007.

16. Holland EJ, et al. Avellino corneal dystrophy. Clinical manifestations and natural history. *Ophthalmology*. 1992;99(10):1564-1568.

17. Jones ST, Zimmerman LE. Histopathologic differentiation of granular, macular, and lattice dystrophies of the cornea. *Am J Ophthalmol*. 1961;51:394-410.

18. SundarRaj N, Barbacci-Tobin E, Howe WE, Robertson SM, Limetti G. Macular corneal dystrophy: immunochemical characterization using monoclonal antibodies. *Invest Ophthalmol Vis Sci*. 1987;28(10):1678-1686.

19. Rodrigues MM, Kruth HS, Krachmer JH, Willis R. Unesterified cholesterol in Schnyder's crystalline dystrophy of the cornea. *Am J Ophthalmol*. 1987;104(2):157-163.

20. Weiss JS, Rodrigues M, Rajagopalan S, Kruth H. Schnyder's corneal dystrophy: clinical, ultrastructural, and histochemical studies. *Ophthalmology*. 1992;99(7):1072-1081. doi:10.1016/S0161-6420(92)31848-2.

21. Witschel H, Fine BS, Grützner P, McTigue JW. Congenital hereditary stromal dystrophy of the cornea. *Arch Ophthalmol*. 1978;96(6):1043-1051.

22. Purcell JJJ, Krachmer JH, Weingeist TA. Fleck corneal dystrophy. *Arch Ophthalmol*. 1977;95:440-444.

23. Dunn SP, Krachmer JH, Ching SST. New findings in posterior amorphous corneal dystrophy. *Arch Ophthalmol*. 1984;102:236-239.

24. Curran RE, Kenyon KR, Green WR. Pre-Descemet's membrane corneal dystrophy. *Am J Ophthalmol*. 1974;77:711-716.

25. Adamis AP, et al. Fuchs' endothelial dystrophy of the cornea. *Surv Ophthalmol*. 1993;38:149-168.

26. Hogan MJ, Wood I, Fine M. Fuchs' endothelial dystrophy of the cornea. *Am J Ophthalmol.* 1974;78:363-383.

27. Waring GO, Rodrigues MM, Laibson PR. Corneal dystrophies. II. Endothelial dystrophies. *Surv Ophthalmol.* 1978;23:147-168.

28. Krachmer JH. Posterior polymorphous corneal dystrophy: a disease characterized by epithelial-like endothelial cells which influence management and prognosis. *Trans Am Ophthalmol Soc.* 1985;83:413-475.

29. Maumenee AE. Congenital hereditary corneal dystrophy. Am J Ophthalmol. 1960;50:1114-1124.

30. Judisch GF, Maumenee IH. Clinical differentiation of recessive congenital hereditary endothelial dystrophy and dominant hereditary endothelial dystrophy. Am J Ophthalmol. 1978;85:606-612.

31. Vithana EN, et al. Mutations in sodium-borate cotransporter SLC4A11 cause recessive congenital hereditary endothelial dystrophy (CHED2). Nat Genet. 2006;38;755-757.

11

Ectasias

KERATOCONUS

KCN is a bilateral disorder in which the central or paracentral cornea bulges and becomes thin, causing progressive irregular astigmatism and sometimes scarring (Figure 11-1).

Signs and Symptoms. Young patients present with progressively increasing astigmatism that becomes difficult to correct with glasses and eventually contacts.

Exams and Tests. Scissoring of the red reflex on retinoscopy can be noted early on. Slit-lamp examination will show central ectasia associated with thinning, stress lines in the deep stroma (Vogt striae), and iron deposits noted around the cone. As the disease progresses, breaks can occur in the Descemet membrane leading to acute corneal edema (hydrops). Topography and tomography can confirm the diagnosis showing inferior steepening and associated corneal thinning.

Treatment. Geared at achieving good vision with glasses or contact lenses. If good vision cannot be achieved, intrastromal ring

Kim T, Daluvoy MB.
The Pocket Guide to Cornea (pp 139–143).
© 2019 SLACK Incorporated.

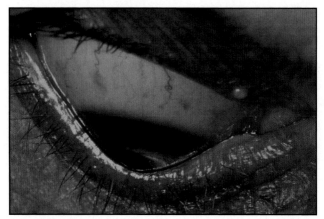

Figure 11-1. Keratoconus. Munson's sign, a V-shaped indentation of the lower eyelid in downgaze, is seen in this slit-lamp photo.

segments (eg, Intacs) can be used to flatten the central cornea. Collagen cross-linking shows promise in halting the progression of ectasia. If/when the condition progresses, a corneal transplant (deep anterior lamellar keratoplasty or penetrating keratoplasty [PKP]) can be performed to improve vision.

PELLUCID MARGINAL DEGENERATION

PMD is an uncommon form of ectasia. Similar to KCN, PMD shows bulging of the cornea and thinning. However, the area of thinning is inferior to the apex of the bulge in PMD, in contrast to KCN, in which thinning coincides with the apex of the cone (Figure 11-2).

Signs and Symptoms. Patients present with progressively increasing astigmatism that becomes difficult to correct with glasses.

Exams and Tests. Slit-lamp examination will show protrusion of the cornea with an area of thinning inferiorly. Topography and

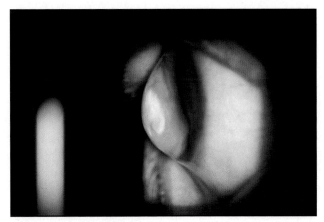

Figure 11-2. Pellucid marginal degeneration. Corneal bulging is seen superior to the area of inferior corneal thinning.

tomography can confirm the diagnosis with its typical "crab-claw" distribution.

Treatment. Geared toward achieving good vision with glasses or contact lenses but can be more difficult in cases of PMD. Owing to the location of the thinning, corneal grafts tend to be large, making success rates lower than in KCN. Collagen cross-linking shows promise in halting the progression of ectasias, but literature on its use with PMD is limited.

KERATOGLOBUS

A very rare, bilateral, uniform thinning and ectasia of the entire cornea that is typically present at birth (Figure 11-3).

Signs and Symptoms. Presents as poor vision needing correction with glasses or contacts.

Exams and Tests. Slit-lamp examination is sufficient to diagnose this condition. Showing uniform thinning and ectasia with a very

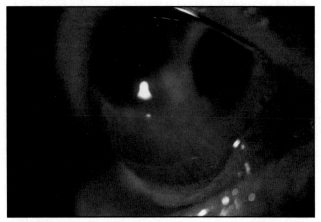

Figure 11-3. Keratoglobus. Peripheral corneal thinning and neovascularization, in addition to a large anterior chamber, are seen.

large anterior chamber, it is often associated with Ehlers-Danlos syndrome so a systemic workup should be conducted if suspected in a child.

Treatment. Prognosis for PKP is poor in these patients because of the thinness of their corneas. Spontaneous rupture has occurred, so patients should be educated about the importance of eye protection from an early age.

POSTREFRACTIVE SURGERY ECTASIA

Corneal ectasia is a rare complication of refractive surgery, particularly given preoperative screening guidelines such as the Ectasia Risk Score System (ERSS) for refractive surgery patient selection. Owing to the greater percentage of corneal tissue altered with LASIK (due to flap creation) than in PRK, postrefractive surgery ectasia is more commonly noted with LASIK than PRK, but remains rare, with a rate at 0.66% in one estimate.

Signs and Symptoms. Postrefractive surgery ectasia typically occurs within 1 to 12 months after refractive surgery. A patient may report a blurring of uncorrected vision in the affected eye, and an inability to completely correct the vision with glasses.

Exams and Tests. Slit-lamp examination may demonstrate corneal thinning and/or protrusion. Corneal topography demonstrates irregular astigmatism, typically with inferior steepening. Corneal tomography may demonstrate posterior float elevation that coincides with the site of maximal thinning on pachymetry mapping.

Treatment. Management is focused primarily on prevention of postrefractive surgery ectasia through careful screening of patients selected for refractive surgery. Risk factors for ectasia include abnormal topography, low residual stromal bed thickness (which can be estimated preoperatively with flap thickness and magnitude of ablation in diopters), younger age, and low preoperative corneal thickness. Risk scores such as the ERSS can help the clinician incorporate these empirically determined risk factors into decision making. Surgeons will typically keep a lower limit of residual stromal bed thickness of 250 µm to 300 µm. This may be increased further to allow for the possible need for future retreatment. If postrefractive surgery ectasia is indicated by diagnostic testing, a hard contact lens can be attempted to address irregular astigmatism. In patients with adequate postoperative corneal thickness, collagen cross-linking may be considered by some clinicians to limit progression of ectasia. If these measures are not applicable or inadequate, anterior lamellar keratoplasty or PKP may become necessary for visual rehabilitation.

BIBLIOGRAPHY

1. Pallikaris IG, Kymionis GD, Astyrakakis NI. Corneal ectasia induced by laser in situ keratomileusis. *J Cataract Refract Surg.* 2001;27(11):1796-802. doi:10.1016/S0886-3350(01)01090-2.

2. Randleman JB, Trattler WB, Stulting RD. Validation of the Ectasia Risk Score System for preoperative laser in situ keratomileusis screening. *Am J Ophthalmol.* 2008;145(5):813-818. doi:10.1016/j.ajo.2007.12.033.

12

Trauma

THERMAL BURNS

Exposure to intense heat can lead to inflammation and scarring of the eyelid, conjunctiva, and cornea (Figure 12-1).

Signs and Symptoms. Eyelid skin burns, conjunctival injection, chemosis, conjunctival defect, cauterized epithelium, scleral thinning or perforation, corneal epithelial defect, corneal haze, iridocyclitis.

Exams and Tests. External and slit-lamp examination should be performed to assess extent of damage.

Treatment. Debridement of devitalized tissue, lubrication, tarsorrhaphy, amniotic membrane grafting, antibiotic ointment, cycloplegic for comfort, cautious use of topical corticosteroids (can help prevent symblepharon formation but can impair corneal healing).

Kim T, Daluvoy MB.
The Pocket Guide to Cornea (pp 145-153).
© 2019 SLACK Incorporated.

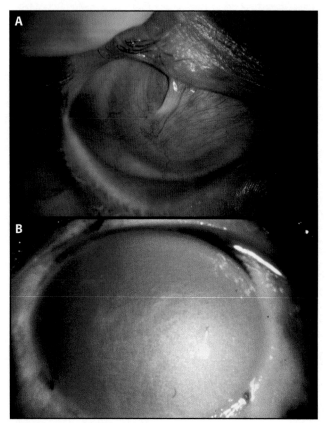

Figure 12-1. Thermal burns. (A) Demonstrates conjunctivalization of the cornea. (B) Demonstrates diffuse corneal haze.

RADIATION

Ultraviolet Radiation

Ultraviolet radiation can induce damage to the corneal epithelium several hours after exposure.

Signs and Symptoms. Foreign body sensation, photophobia, punctate epithelial erosions particularly in interpalpebral region.

Exams and Tests. Slit-lamp examination with fluorescein staining should be performed.

Treatment. Generally self-limited. Symptoms can be managed with preservative-free artificial tears, ointment, and cycloplegic drops.

Ionizing Radiation

Exposure to ionizing radiation such as x-rays, radioisotopes, and nuclear explosions may lead to tissue destruction through direct cytotoxicity, DNA mutations, and radiation damage to blood vessels leading to ischemia.

Signs and Symptoms. Chemosis, conjunctival scarring, punctate corneal erosions, radiation necrosis, poor wound healing.

Exams and Tests. External and slit-lamp examination should be performed to assess extent of damage.

Treatment. Artificial tears, antibiotic ointment, bandage contact lens, tarsorrhaphy, conjunctival flap, amniotic membrane graft, limbal stem cell transplant.

CHEMICAL INJURIES

Alkali Burns

Alkali compounds can cause rapid and extensive destruction because of their ability to readily penetrate the corneal stroma.

Signs and Symptoms. Conjunctival injection, chemosis, corneal epithelial defects, corneal haze, limbal ischemia, corneal melt or perforation with damage to iris or lens, iridocyclitis.

Exams and Tests. External and slit-lamp examination should be performed to assess extent of damage.

Treatment. Immediate and copious irrigation with saline or tap water until pH neutralizes to 7 (wait 5 to 10 minutes after irrigation to retest pH) and removal of toxic particulate materials or foreign bodies from fornices. For mild cases, can use preservative-free artificial tears, topical antibiotic ointment, cycloplegic and intraocular pressure-lowering agents as needed; oral doxycycline and topical acetylcysteine to decrease collagenase activity; high-dose oral vitamin C; and consider topical steroids if significant inflammation (but can increase risk of corneal melt). For severe cases, topical sodium citrate 10%, debridement of necrotic tissue, consider bandage contact lens, amniotic membrane graft, tarsorrhaphy, cyanoacrylate glue or corneal patch graft for perforation. May require limbal stem cell transplantation, keratoplasty, or keratoprosthesis.

Acid Burns

Acids also cause burns but to a lesser extent than alkalis because of the natural buffering ability of tissues, and the precipitation of proteins acts as barrier to further penetration. Findings and management are similar to that of alkali burns.

Medication Toxicity

Compounds contained in topical ophthalmic medications can lead to epithelial keratopathy. Common offending agents include benzalkonium chloride, aminoglycosides, antivirals, glaucoma medications, and topical anesthetics.

Signs and Symptoms. Foreign body sensation, conjunctival injection, conjunctival or corneal punctate epithelial erosions, papillary reaction, follicular response, sterile infiltrate in severe cases.

Exams and Tests. Slit-lamp examination with fluorescein staining and inspection of conjunctiva should be performed.

Treatment. Removal of potential offending agent, lubrication with preservative-free artificial tears or ointment.

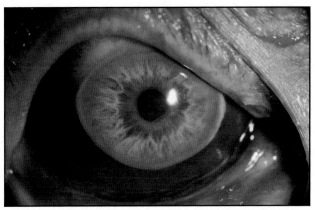

Figure 12-2. Subconjunctival hemorrhage. Blood is present in the subconjunctival space.

VEGETATION INJURIES

Any injury to the ocular surface caused by vegetable matter.

Signs and Symptoms. Foreign body sensation, conjunctival injection, epithelial defects, stromal infiltrate.

Exams and Tests. Slit-lamp examination with fluorescein staining should be performed, as well as sweeping of fornices and eversion of lids to identify foreign bodies.

Treatment. Immediate irrigation and removal of foreign bodies, topical cycloplegics, and prophylactic antibiotics. Avoid topical steroids as they can predispose to fungal infections.

MECHANICAL TRAUMA

Subconjunctival Hemorrhage

Blood under the conjunctiva, which can be caused by trauma, valsalva maneuvers, anticoagulation, or be idiopathic (Figure 12-2).

Signs and Symptoms. Painless red eye (often sectoral).

Exams and Tests. If history of trauma, rule out penetrating injury. If recurrent, consider systemic workup to evaluate for bleeding diathesis, hypertension, and diabetes mellitus.

Treatment. Reassurance that condition will self-resolve in 1 to 2 weeks.

Conjunctival Laceration

Laceration of the conjunctiva usually caused by trauma.

Signs and Symptoms. Redness, foreign body sensation, pain.

Exams and Tests. Slit-lamp examination should be performed using cotton swab or sterile forceps to rule out deeper injury. Consider conjunctival peritomy in operating room if unable to determine extent of injury at slit-lamp examination.

Treatment. Antibiotic ointment for comfort as most conjunctival lacerations will self-heal. If laceration is large (> 1.5 cm), consider suturing with 8-0 Vicryl.

Conjunctival Foreign Body

Foreign bodies can become lodged onto the conjunctiva, most commonly in the inferior fornix or underneath the upper eyelid.

Signs and Symptoms. Foreign body sensation, redness, tearing.

Treatment. Search for foreign body by everting upper eyelid, sweep superior and inferior fornices, irrigate fornices, fluorescein staining to identify corneal abrasions caused by foreign body embedded under eyelid.

Treatment. Removal of foreign body with sterile jewelers or hypodermic needle. Leave deeply buried foreign bodies unless vegetative or proinflammatory.

Corneal Foreign Body

Foreign body embedded in the cornea (Figure 12-3).

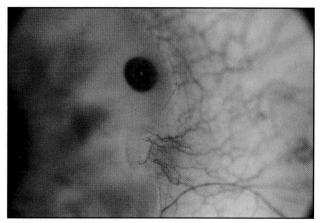

Figure 12-3. Corneal foreign body. A metallic corneal foreign body is seen with a rust ring.

Signs and Symptoms. Pain, foreign body sensation, redness, tearing.

Exams and Tests. Slit-lamp examination should be performed to identify foreign body and depth, Seidel testing to assess if perforation has occurred.

Treatment. If superficial, gentle removal with sterile jewelers forceps or cotton tip. Removal in operating room if extension into anterior chamber. If rust ring has formed from a metallic foreign body, removal with hypodermic needle or corneal burr, taking care to minimize tissue disruption (to reduce scarring) and avoid perforation. Treat underlying corneal abrasion.

Corneal Abrasion

A corneal abrasion is a corneal epithelial defect that can be a result of trauma, exposure, infection, or inflammation.

Signs and Symptoms. Pain, foreign body sensation, tearing, photophobia.

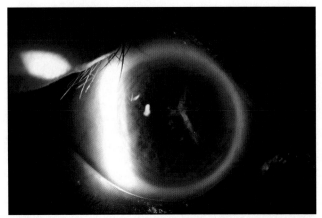

Figure 12-4. Corneal laceration. A corneal laceration reapposed with 10-0 nylon sutures is seen.

Exams and Tests. Slit-lamp examination with fluorescein staining should be performed, as well as eversion of eyelids to rule out foreign body.

Treatment. Antibiotic ointment, topical cycloplegic. Consider debridement of loose epithelium to promote better healing and topical nonsteroidal inflammatory agents or bandage contact lens for pain.

Corneal Laceration

Partial or full-thickness corneal defect, usually as a result of trauma (Figure 12-4).

Signs and Symptoms. Pain, gush of fluid, shallow anterior chamber, Seidel-positive corneal wound, pupil distortion, prolapse of intraocular contents, violation of lens capsule, poor visual acuity.

Exams and Tests. Complete systemic and ocular examination to identify extent of trauma, Seidel test, noncontrast computed tomography with orbital cuts to evaluate for intraocular foreign body. Avoid performing any maneuvers that apply pressure to the eye, such as tonometry, gonioscopy, ultrasound, forced duction testing, or scleral depression.

Treatment. Protective shield, pain control, antiemetics, prophylactic systemic antibiotics (fluoroquinolones have best ocular penetration), tetanus prophylaxis. Surgical repair should take place within 24 hours with primary goal of globe closure. If there is a self-sealed wound, repair may be unnecessary or delayed. Restoration of vision is a secondary goal (either at time of primary or subsequent surgery). If extensive damage with no visual potential, consider enucleation (either primary or secondary within 14 days) to prevent sympathetic ophthalmia.

BIBLIOGRAPHY

1. Wagoner MD. Chemical injuries of the eye: current concepts in pathophysiology and therapy. *Surv Ophthalmol.* 1997;41(4):275-313.
2. Westekemper H, Figueiredo FC, Siah WF, Wagner N, Steuhl KP, Meller D. Clinical outcomes of amniotic membrane transplantation in the management of acute ocular chemical injury. *Br J Ophthalmol.* 2017;101(2):103-107. doi: 10.1136/bjophthalmol-2015-308037.
3. Vora GK, Haddadin R, Chodosh J. Management of corneal lacerations and perforations. *Int Ophthalmol Clin.* 2013;53(4):1-10. doi: 10.1097/IIO.0b013e3182a12c08.
4. Mannis MJ, Holland EJ, eds. *Cornea.* 4th ed. Edinburgh, Scotland: Elsevier Inc; 2016.

13

Procedures and Surgeries

CORNEAL TRANSPLANTATION

Penetrating Keratoplasty

PKP refers to transplantation of a donor cornea to replace the full thickness of a host cornea (Figure 13-1A).

Indications. PKP can be performed for a wide variety of reasons, including corneal opacification, irregular corneal shape, reinforcement of a thinned cornea, and to address corneal infection.

Preoperative Evaluation. Evaluation of the PKP surgical candidate should include a complete history and ophthalmic examination, including dilated fundus examination (to the extent possible given corneal pathology). History should include coexisting and prior ocular conditions and prior surgeries (including prior corneal transplants). Intraocular pressure (IOP) should be noted and controlled prior to surgery. Lens status should be identified, as phakic patients will require special care to avoid intraoperative lens disruption. The nature of the corneal pathology will affect

Kim T, Daluvoy MB.
The Pocket Guide to Cornea (pp 155-170).
© 2019 SLACK Incorporated.

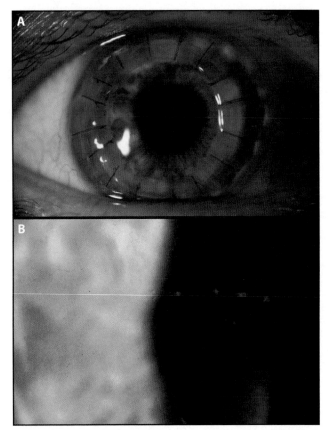

Figure 13-1. Penetrating keratoplasty. (A) A penetrating keratoplasty graft secured with interrupted 10-0 nylon sutures. (B) A rejection line is seen on the endothelium.

prognosis for the graft. The presence or absence of corneal neovascularization should be noted and addressed if possible. The size, shape, and location of graft required should be identified or estimated preoperatively.

Postoperative Evaluation. In the early postoperative period, evaluation should include checking for epithelial defect, infection, and signs of graft rejection (including rejection lines (Figure 13-1B), anterior chamber cells, keratic precipitates, neovascularization, and edema). Late postoperative evaluation is focused on minimizing astigmatism through suture management and avoidance of graft rejection.

Complications. Potential intraoperative complications may include lens disruption in phakic patients, loss of intraocular contents due to posterior pressure, and suprachoroidal hemorrhage (which may also lead to loss of intraocular contents). Postoperative complications include wound leak, persistent epithelial defect, elevated IOP, anterior synechiae formation, infection, and graft failure or rejection.

Anterior Lamellar Keratoplasty

ALK refers to a set of procedures in which a corneal stromal pathology is addressed by replacing the anterior cornea with the same-thickness donor tissue. This can be considered only when the endothelium is normal. The most common form is deep anterior lamellar keratoplasty (DALK), in which the entire stroma is removed and only the Descemet membrane (DM) and endothelium remain.

Indications. ALK can be performed to address corneal stromal opacification and/or thinning when deeper stroma and/or endothelium is normal.

Preoperative Evaluation. Complete ophthalmic history and examination should be performed. The status of the corneal endothelium and DM should be evaluated, including assessment for breaks in the DM and adequacy of endothelial cell function.

Postoperative Evaluation. Check for epithelial defect and infection. Good approximation of the donor and host tissue should be noted. Late postoperative evaluation is focused on minimizing astigmatism through suture management and avoidance of graft rejection.

Complications. The most common intraoperative complication of DALK is perforation or rupture of DM, and it can happen at any of several steps during the procedure, but can easily be converted to a PKP if needed.

Endothelial Keratoplasty

Endothelial keratoplasty (EK) refers to a set of procedures used to address endothelial dysfunction by replacing abnormal DM and endothelial cells with partial-thickness donor tissue. The 2 most common forms of EK are Descemet-stripping endothelial keratoplasty (DSEK; Figure 13-2A) and Descemet membrane endothelial keratoplasty (DMEK; Figure 13-2B). DSEK involves replacement of host DM and endothelium with donor partial-thickness stroma, DM, and endothelium. DMEK involves replacement of host DM and endothelium with donor DM and endothelium. DMEK offers improved visual acuity, decreased rate of rejection, and faster visual recover in comparison to DSEK, but is a more technically complex surgery and has a higher rate of graft detachment than DSEK.

Indications. EK can be performed to address endothelial dystrophies such as Fuchs' endothelial dystrophy, postsurgical conditions such as pseudophakic bullous keratopathy, trauma from anterior chamber implants, and failed corneal grafts (including PKP and prior EK).

Preoperative Evaluation. Complete ophthalmic history and examination should be performed. Serial corneal pachymetry measurements can be utilized to assess progression of corneal edema. Specular microscopy can be used to evaluate for endothelial cell polymegathism, pleomorphism, and density reduction. Phakic patients and patients with glaucoma drainage devices may be better candidates for DSEK than DMEK because of the relative ease of graft manipulation intraoperatively. Patients with cataracts may be considered for a "triple" procedure, involving cataract removal, lens implantation, and EK in the same operation.

Postoperative Evaluation. In the early postoperative period, patients should be evaluated for the positioning and adherence of the

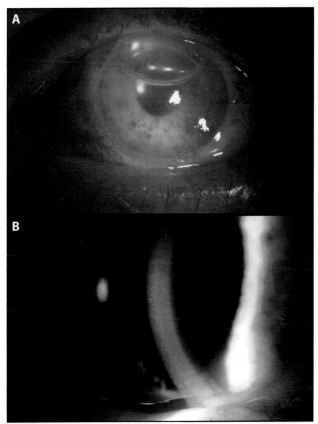

Figure 13-2. Endothelial keratoplasty. (A) The DSEK graft is pictured on post-operative day 1 with an air bubble in the anterior chamber to help the graft adhere to the host. (B) The DMEK graft (red arrow) is attached with the slit beam, showing that the cornea is compact without any edema.

graft, the anterior chamber gas bubble, and IOP. Late evaluations are focused on corneal clearance and monitoring for graft rejection.

Complications. Possible complications include graft dislocation or detachment, development of pupillary block due to a large gas bubble, early graft decompensation due to intraoperative trauma, interface deposits, refractive changes (typically hyperopic shift), and graft rejection.

Ocular Surface Reconstruction

Phototherapeutic Keratectomy. PTK refers to the use of an excimer laser to "photoablate" corneal surface tissue in a controlled manner for the purpose of addressing corneal pathology.

Indications. PTK is utilized in the treatment of superficial corneal dystrophies (including epithelial basement membrane dystrophy), corneal surface irregularities (such as Salzmann nodular degeneration), and corneal opacifications.

Preoperative Evaluation. Complete ophthalmic history and examination should be performed. Corneal topography can be utilized to identify the extent of surface irregularity. Assessment of the depth of corneal pathology is essential, as it is ideal to maintain a residual corneal thickness of 350 μm or more after ablation to reduce the risk of corneal ectasia. This assessment can be performed by slit-lamp examination, anterior segment optical coherence tomography (OCT), or confocal microscopy.

Postoperative Evaluation. Early postoperative evaluation is focused on monitoring healing of the epithelium and pain management. Later evaluations are focused on monitoring for development of anterior stromal haze, which may be treated prophylactically with intraoperative mitomycin C or postoperatively with steroids. For corneal dystrophies treated with PTK, evaluation for recurrence is warranted.

Complications. Pain, poor healing of corneal epithelium, and development of anterior stromal haze are the most common adverse effects of PTK. Nonuniform ablation can lead to worsening irregularity of the corneal surface or induced refractive error. Excessive ablation can lead to corneal ectasia. For patients with a history of herpetic disease, reactivation may also occur after PTK, often warranting prophylactic antiviral therapy.

Amniotic Membrane Transplantation

AMT refers to the affixing of amniotic membrane (the innermost layer of the placenta) to the ocular surface with glue or sutures for the purpose of promoting epithelial healing and/or reducing ocular surface inflammation. The amniotic membrane consists of an epithelial layer, a basement membrane, and a stromal matrix. It has been found to reduce proteolytic activity and suppress production of proinflammatory cytokines. The membrane naturally reabsorbs over time. There are 2 commercially available types of amniotic membrane grafts: freeze-dried and frozen.

Indications. AMT is utilized for the treatment of nonhealing epithelial defects (such as in neurotrophic keratopathy), for the promotion of reepithelialization after corneal or conjunctival surgery, and inflammatory corneal thinning. It is also frequently utilized to promote healing of corneal burns and acute Stevens-Johnson syndrome. Although it contains no stem cells itself, AMT is utilized in patients with limbal stem cell deficiency to promote reepithelialization after limbal stem cell transplantation or superficial keratectomy.

Preoperative Evaluation. Complete ophthalmic history and examination should be performed. Fluorescein staining can aid in the visualization of persistent epithelial defects. Examination of the eyelid architecture and presence of symblepharon will help guide the size and type of amniotic membrane graft required.

Postoperative Evaluation. Postoperatively, the resorption of the transplanted amniotic membrane is monitored, as well as the underlying condition.

Complications. Complications of AMT are rare; there is no risk of rejection.

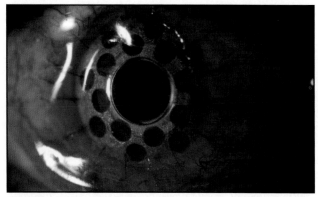

Figure 13-3. Boston type 1 keratoprosthesis. The optic is held in place by donor tissue and a titanium back plate.

Keratoprosthesis

K-Pro refers to a variety of artificial corneas utilized to treat patients who are either not candidates for corneal transplantation or have already failed corneal transplantation (Figure 13-3).

Indications. While several forms of K-Pro currently exist and are under development, the Boston K-Pro is most commonly used. Two types of the Boston K-Pro are available: Type I has broad application to patients with corneal opacification, while type II (implanted through the closed eyelid) is indicated for patients with severe keratinizing dry eye. The type I Boston K-Pro is often utilized for patients with multiple prior corneal transplant failures, chemical or thermal injury, and severe autoimmune disorders (such as Stevens-Johnson syndrome) and other limbal stem cell diseases.

Preoperative Evaluation. Complete ophthalmic history and examination should be performed. B-scan and anterior segment OCT may be needed because of poor visibility through an opaque cornea. The lens status of the patient is important to determine what power K-Pro to implant. Because of the possibility of developing vision-threatening complications such as glaucoma and retinal detachment after K-Pro implantation, the necessity of surgery should be carefully weighed, particularly in patients in whom the fellow eye is adequate for visual function. If glaucoma is already present or suspected, a drainage device may be needed at the time of surgery.

Postoperative Evaluation. Typical postoperative evaluations should involve slit-lamp examination, IOP measurement (by palpation or scleral pneumotonometry), Seidel testing, optic nerve evaluation, and examination of the retinal periphery. Ongoing careful monitoring for glaucoma, infection, or sterile inflammation is recommended.

Complications. K-Pro complications include development or worsening of glaucoma, retinal detachment, development of a retroprosthetic membrane, sterile vitritis, endophthalmitis, and corneal melt around the prosthesis. At some centers, prophylactic placement of glaucoma drainage devices and 360° peripheral retinal laser are performed prophylactically because of these concerns.

Limbal Stem Cell Transplantation

Limbal stem cell transplantation refers to a wide variety of techniques utilized to treat deficiency of limbal epithelial stem cells. Techniques include conjunctival limbal autograft, living related conjunctival limbal allograft, keratolimbal allograft, simple limbal epithelial transplant, and cultivated limbal epithelial transplant.

Indications. Indicated for patients with evidence of limbal stem cell deficiency, which can occur in the setting of contact lens wear, autoimmune disease, chemical or thermal burns, severe prior infection, congenital conditions, and prior ocular surgery.

Preoperative Evaluation. Complete ophthalmic history and examination should be performed. Fluorescein staining may highlight a whorled epithelial pattern in some cases. In deciding on an appropriate therapeutic approach, the status of the fellow eye is an important factor, as bilateral disease precludes the use of an autograft. The tear film should be assessed, as insufficient lubrication will impair graft survival. The presence or absence of systemic disease (such as uncontrolled diabetes, hepatic dysfunction, and renal insufficiency) is also important, as the need for systemic immunosuppression with many forms of limbal stem cell transplantation may preclude systemically ill patients from undergoing transplantation.

Postoperative Evaluation. Postoperative evaluation is focused on the vascularization of the graft, assessment for evidence of rejection, and reepithelialization of the cornea.

Complications. Potential complications include graft misalignment, acute rejection, chronic rejection, and infection due to chronic immunosuppression.

STROMAL MICROPUNCTURE

A treatment option for patients with recurrent corneal erosions, stromal micropuncture involves creation of adhesions between the epithelium and anterior stroma with multiple shallow penetrations of the anterior cornea with a needle (often 20, 23, or 25 gauge).

Indications. Stromal micropuncture is performed for patients with recurrent epithelial erosions outside the visual axis refractory to conservative management such as lubrication and bandage contact lenses.

Preoperative Evaluation. Complete ophthalmic history and examination should be performed. Fluorescein staining can aid in the visualization of areas warranting treatment.

Postoperative Evaluation. Patients should be monitored for development of new epithelial erosion outside the treatment area or recurrence within the treatment area.

Complications. Loss of control of penetration depth with the needle may result in deep stromal scarring or full-thickness penetration of the cornea. This can generally be avoided with careful positioning and use of a standardized needle.

CORNEAL GLUING

Typically utilizing cyanoacrylate or fibrin formulations, corneal gluing involves the application of an adhesive for the purpose of temporarily sealing a perforated cornea or reinforcing a severely thinned cornea. The glue can be applied with any of a variety of techniques, including careful painting of the defect using a 30-gauge needle and covering with a bandage contact lens.

Indications. Corneal gluing may be utilized as a temporizing measure for corneal perforation or severe thinning due to trauma, infection, or inflammation.

Preoperative Evaluation. Complete ophthalmic history and examination should be performed. Seidel testing will confirm a leak. Evaluation should include identification of the cause and extent of the corneal defect

Postoperative Evaluation. After completion of gluing, eyes with corneal perforation should be evaluated for reformation of the anterior chamber, indicating adequate sealing of the defect.

Complications. Excessive application of glue can lead to substantial irritation. Displacement of the glue plug may also occur.

REFRACTIVE SURGERY

Laser-Assisted in situ Keratomileusis

Laser-assisted in situ keratomileusis, better known as LASIK, alters the corneal curvature to change the refractive power of the eye. It involves the creation of an intrastromal corneal flap with either a microkeratome or a femtosecond laser, reflection of the flap, use of an excimer laser to reshape the residual stromal bed, and finally replacement of the corneal flap.

Indications. LASIK can be performed for correction of refractive error in patients with a stable refraction between –12.0 diopters and +6.0 diopters as well as astigmatism.

Preoperative Evaluation. Complete ophthalmic history and examination should be performed. Age is an important factor as stability of refraction increases the likelihood of a lasting treatment effect. Presbyopic patients may consider treatment options such as monovision (one eye set for near vision and one set for distance vision). Pupil size measurement, ocular dominance testing, and dry eye testing are performed. Manifest and cycloplegic refraction, corneal topography, and corneal tomography are critical. Refraction indicates whether myopic or hyperopic ablation will be performed, topography indicates the presence of regular or irregular astigmatism, and tomography provides indication of corneal thickness. Any irregularities on testing must be critically evaluated to rule out those at risk for postoperative ectasia. Wavefront analysis may also be performed to better understand the patient's higher-order aberrations and allow for their correction with a customized ablation pattern.

Postoperative Evaluation. Visual acuity is tested and manifest refraction may be obtained as needed. Slit-lamp examination is performed, taking particular note of flap positioning and the flap-bed interface for any irregularities such as striae or cells.

Complications. Potential intraoperative complications include an incomplete, buttonholed, thin, or free flap and decentration during ablation. Potential postoperative complications include flap displacement or striae, epithelial ingrowth (Figure 13-4), diffuse lamellar keratitis, infectious keratitis, corneal ectasia (see Postrefractive Surgery Ectasia), and regression of treatment effect. In addition, dry eye is a potential postoperative adverse effect.

Photorefractive Keratectomy

PRK is a form of excimer laser surface ablation used to treat refractive error without the creation of an intrastromal flap. It is often employed in patients who are highly active and would be at risk of traumatic flap dislocation, patients with borderline corneal thickness who would potentially be at risk for post-LASIK ectasia, patients with dry eye, and patients who have experienced LASIK flap complications.

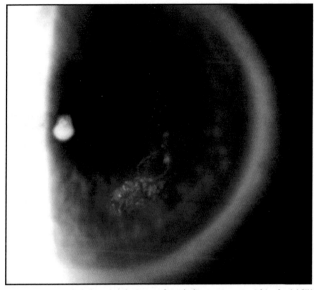

Figure 13-4. Epithelial ingrowth. Rests of epithelium are seen within the LASIK flap interface.

Indications. PRK is indicated for the correction of refractive errors between –10 diopters and +4 diopters. Reasons for considering PRK over LASIK are discussed above and are highly surgeon dependent.

Preoperative Evaluation. See LASIK.

Postoperative Evaluation. Visual acuity is tested and manifest refraction may be obtained. Slit-lamp examination is performed, taking note of epithelial healing and assessing for development of anterior stromal haze.

Complications. Decentration of ablation is a potential intraoperative complication. Potential postoperative complications include dry eye, corneal ectasia (see Postrefractive Surgery Ectasia), anterior stromal haze, and regression of treatment effect.

MANAGEMENT OF CORNEAL ECTASIA

Corneal Cross-Linking

CXL is a procedure used to enhance the structural integrity of the cornea through the formation of chemical bonds between adjacent collagen fibrils. It involves the application of a photosensitizing agent (typically riboflavin) and the exposure of the cornea to ultraviolet light.

Indications. CXL is indicated for unstable keratoconus, postrefractive surgery ectasia, and other forms of ectasia.

Preoperative Evaluation. Complete ophthalmic history and examination should be performed. Serial refraction, corneal topography, and corneal tomography are all helpful in assessing the rapidity of progression and overall severity of corneal ectatic changes.

Postoperative Evaluation. Slit-lamp examination is performed to monitor epithelial healing and presence of haze. Refraction, corneal topography, and corneal tomography may be repeated at regular intervals to assess for deceleration of ectasia progression.

Complications. Potential complications include stromal edema, stromal haze, and corneal inflammation or infection.

Intrastromal Corneal Ring Segments

ICRS are poly(methyl methacrylate) (PMMA) implants placed in the corneal periphery to flatten the central cornea and provide biomechanical support to the corneal tissue (Figure 13-5). Today, channels for placement of ICRS are typically made utilizing a femtosecond laser.

Indications. ICRS can be used for the correction of low myopia as well as correction of irregular astigmatism in corneal ectasias. The central flattening effect and biomechanical support have led to ICRS being used commonly in patients with keratoconus.

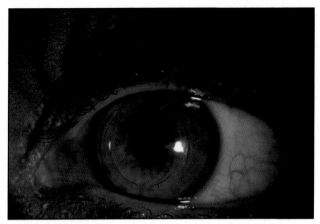

Figure 13-5. Intrastromal corneal ring segments. Paired ring segments are seen oriented at 90 degrees.

Preoperative Evaluation. Complete ophthalmic history and examination should be performed. Refraction, corneal topography, and corneal tomography are typically performed. This testing is essential in the selection of the type, depth, and location of the implants to be placed.

Postoperative Evaluation. Visual acuity is tested and manifest refraction may be obtained. Slit-lamp examination is performed, taking note of implant positioning and incision closure.

Complications. Potential intraoperative complications include anterior or posterior perforation during channel creation and decentration. Potential postoperative complications include infectious keratitis, incisional gaping, implant migration, intrastromal deposits, and glare.

BIBLIOGRAPHY

1. Melles GRJ, Lander F, Nieuwendaal C. Sutureless, posterior lamellar keratoplasty: A case report of a modified technique. *Cornea.* 2002;21:325-327. doi:10.1097/00003226-200204000-00018.

2. Lu P, Li L, Mukaida N, Zhang X. Alkali-induced corneal neovascularization is independent of CXCR2-mediated neutrophil infiltration. *Cornea.* 2007;26:199-206. doi:10.1097/01.ico.0000248385.16896.34.

3. Melles GRJ. Posterior lamellar keratoplasty: DLEK to DSEK to DMEK. *Cornea.* 2006;25:879-881. doi:10.1097/01.ico.0000243962.60392.4f.

4. Di Zazzo A, Kheirkhah A, Abud TB, Goyal S, Dana R. Management of high-risk corneal transplantation. *Surv Ophthalmol.* 2017;62:816-827. doi:10.1016/j.survophthal.2016.12.010.

5. Choi JA, Lee MA, Kim MS. Long-term outcomes of penetrating keratoplasty in keratoconus: analysis of the factors associated with final visual acuities. *Int J Ophthalmol.* 2014;7:517-521. doi:10.3980/j.issn.2222-3959.2014.03.24.

6. Pedrotti E, Passilongo M, Fasolo A, Ficial S, Ferrari S, Marchini G. Refractive outcomes of penetrating keratoplasty and deep anterior lamellar keratoplasty in fellow eyes for keratoconus. *Int Ophthalmol.* 2017;37:911-919. doi:10.1007/s10792-016-0350-0.

7. Jirsova K, Jones GLA. Amniotic membrane in ophthalmology: properties, preparation, storage and indications for grafting—a review. *Cell Tissue Bank.* 2017;18:193-204. doi:10.1007/s10561-017-9618-5.

8. Yin J, Jurkunas U. Limbal stem cell transplantation and complications. *Semin Ophthalmol.* 2018;33:134-141. doi:10.1080/08820538.2017.1353834.

9. Aravena C, Yu F, Aldave AJ. Long-term visual outcomes, complications, and retention of the boston type I keratoprosthesis. *Cornea.* 2018;37:3-10. doi:10.1097/ICO.0000000000001405.

10. Mohammadpour M, Masoumi A, Mirghorbani M, Shahraki K, Hashemi H. Updates on corneal collagen cross-linking: Indications, techniques and clinical outcomes. *J Curr Ophthalmol.* 2017;29:235-247. doi:10.1016/j.joco.2017.07.003.

11. Chua D, Htoon HM, Lim L, et al. Eighteen-year prospective audit of LASIK outcomes for myopia in 53 731 eyes. *Br J Ophthalmol.* 2018;24:bjophthalmol-2018-312587. doi:10.1136/bjophthalmol-2018-312587.

Financial Disclosures

Dr. Melissa B. Daluvoy has no financial or proprietary interest in the materials presented herein.

Dr. Michelle J. Kim has no financial or proprietary interest in the materials presented herein.

Dr. Terry Kim is a consultant for Aerie Pharmaceuticals, Alcon/Novartis, Allergan/Actavis, Avedro, Avellino Labs, Bausch + Lomb/Valeant, Blephex, CoDa/Ocunexus Therapeutics, CorneaGen, Johnson & Johnson Vision, Kala Pharmaceuticals, NovaBay Pharmaceuticals, Ocular Therapeutix, Omeros, Powervision, Presbyopia Therapies, Shire, Simple Contacts, TearLab, and Zeiss and has ownership in Avellino Labs, CorneaGen, Kala Pharmaceuticals, NovaBay Pharmaceuticals, Ocular Therapeutix, Omeros, and Simple Contacts.

Dr. Nambi Nallasamy has no financial or proprietary interest in the materials presented herein.

Index